Constitutional Oncogenetics

To my colleagues and friends from the oncogenetics centers from whom I have learned so much:

Prof. Yves-Jean Bignon and his team,
Centre Jean-Perrin, Clermont-Ferrand;

Dr. Olivier Caron and his team,
Institut Gustave Roussy, Paris;

Dr. Dominique Stoppa Lyonnet,
Dr. Chrystelle Colas and
Dr. Emmanuelle Fourme,
Institut Curie, Paris

SCIENCES

Health and Society, Field Director – Bruno Salgues

Health Changes and Resistances, Subject Head – Bruno Salgues

Constitutional Oncogenetics

Noureddine Boukhatem

iSTE

WILEY

First published 2021 in Great Britain and the United States by ISTE Ltd and John Wiley & Sons, Inc.

ISTE Ltd
27-37 St George's Road
London SW19 4EU
UK

www.iste.co.uk

John Wiley & Sons, Inc.
111 River Street
Hoboken, NJ 07030
USA

www.wiley.com

Library of Congress Control Number: 2020946632

British Library Cataloguing-in-Publication Data
A CIP record for this book is available from the British Library
ISBN 978-1-78945-016-3

ERC code:
LS2 Genetics, 'Omics', Bioinformatics and Systems Biology
LS2_5 Epigenetics and gene regulation
LS7 Applied Medical Technologies, Diagnostics, Therapies and Public Health
LS7_2 Genetic tools for medical diagnosis

MIX
Paper from responsible sources
FSC® C013604

Contents

Foreword

I know Professor Noureddine Boukhatem from Mohamed I University in Morocco well, and I have been able to appreciate during his visits, since 2017, to my oncogenetics department at the Centre Jean-Perrin in Clermont-Ferrand his human qualities, his commitment and his enthusiasm for oncogenetics. A "Tour de France" of major oncogenetic consultations has enabled him to have an informed and multidisciplinary view of modern oncogenetics.

Oncogenetics is defined as the management of families presenting a suspected hereditary risk of cancer, which is considered to be the cancer risk factor with by far the highest predictive value. The discovery of the first hereditary cancer risk genes in the late 1980s (TP53 and RB1 genes) provided doctors with a diagnostic tool that was essential to the practice of oncogenetics. The high predictive value of these genetic tests enables the physician to implement screening measures for individuals and families at high risk of cancer in order to improve the prognosis when cancer occurs, but also to implement preventive measures for high-risk cancers whenever possible in order to reduce their incidence.

Oncogenetics came into existence about 30 years ago in a few countries, including France, which in 1991 created the Génétique et Cancer (Genetics and Cancer) group, which structured the national organization of oncogenetics through the implementation of the first consultations in Clermont-Ferrand, then in Lyon and then in Paris. It was not until 2002–2003 that the first cancer plan led to the creation of the Institut national du cancer (French National Cancer Institute), which then officially supported oncogenetic activities, first in the molecular diagnosis laboratory, then in consultation and then in the monitoring of people at high risk of cancer. From this support, a territorial network was set up to provide effective care for families at high risk of cancer. France has thus become a model of organization at the national level of oncogenetics.

Oncogenetics has developed mainly in Europe and North America. Unfortunately, this discipline remains elementary or reserved for a fortuitous and educated elite in many countries, particularly in Asia and Africa. This is why Professor Noureddine Boukhatem's approach to writing a book on oncogenetics is valuable and useful for the medical community. He has produced an encyclopedic work with a concise presentation and an extensive bibliography, highly useful as a reference. This work is thus strongly recommended for oncogenetic doctors or students who are going to practice medical genetics.

Yves-Jean BIGNON
Director of the oncogenetics department
Centre Jean-Perrin in Clermont-Ferrand
October 2020

Introduction

This book offers a concise and precise state of the art in the field of genetic predisposition to cancer. It provides an up-to-date overview of a field that is still in the process of maturing. The emphasis is on clinical aspects in relation to the practice of oncogenetic counseling as undertaken in France based on my experience in three oncogenetic services (the Centre Jean-Perrin in Clermont-Ferrand, the Institut Gustave-Roussy and the Institut Curie in Paris).

In Parts 1 and 2, which are the focus of this book, we catalogue the genetic predisposition syndromes for cancer. We deal with the syndromes in order of frequency, as deduced from statistics on patients and their relatives carrying a genetic alteration predisposing to cancer and identified in 2016 by the various accredited centers reported by the Institut National du Cancer.

Thus, in Part 1, we start with breast/ovarian cancer predisposition syndrome and Lynch syndrome, of which the suspicion of their presence is the primary reason for oncogenetic consultations. Genetic alterations predisposing to these two syndromes identified in index patients and their relatives in 2016 in France represented 67% of all genetic predispositions to cancer (breast/ovary 53% and Lynch 14%). We then deal with the other syndromes for which the percentage of genetic alterations identified as predisposing them is greater than 1%. In Part 2, we describe the syndromes for which the percentage of genetic alterations predisposing them is less than 1%.

DEFINITION.– *The term* index case *(patient zero) is used to refer to the first person in an outbreak to have been infected with a pathogen. Here, the index case or index patient is the first person in a family where a genetic abnormality (mutation in the broadest sense) has been detected.*

DEFINITION.– *The term* relative *refers to a person who has a family (blood) relation to the index case.*

DEFINITION.– *The term* syndrome *refers to a group of several symptoms characteristic of a specific disease, constituting a recognizable clinical entity and attributable to a certain cause.*

DEFINITION.– *The term* genetic predisposition *refers to an increased likelihood or probability of developing a particular disease due to the presence of one or more mutations in the gene and/or a family history indicating an increased risk of the disease. It is also known as* genetic susceptibility.

In this book, we consider the syndromes of genetic predisposition to cancers that were diagnosed in France in 2016 (see Table I.1). These syndromes are classified here (see Table I.2) according to statistics on index patients and their relatives carrying a genetic alteration predisposing to cancer, identified in the various accredited centers in France in 2016.

The national organization of oncogenetics in France, under the aegis of the INCa, is a unique and efficient model enabling complete care of the families concerned. Figure I.1, reproduced from the INCa report cited above, gives a summary of the path of index patients and their relatives through the oncogenetic circuit.

Predispositions	Genes	AR	IC+	REL+	Total
Breast ovarian syndrome (including isolated ovarian cancers)	BRCA1	/	893	1,280	4,356
	BRCA2	/	777	1,165	
	PALB2	/	64	51	
	RAD51	/	16	8	
	Other	/	12	0	
Lynch syndrome	MLH1	/	128	203	1,148
	MSH2	/	163	236	
	MSH6	/	116	134	
	PMS2	/	54	93	
	EPCAM	/	6	10	
	Other*	/	1	4	

Predispositions	Genes	AR	IC+	REL+	Total
Familial adenomatous polyposis	APC	/	128	148	528
	MUTYH	BI	64	20	
		MONO	72	86	
	POLE	/	4	4	
	POLD1	/	1	0	
	NTHL1	BI	1	0	
		MONO	0	0	
Hereditary diffuse gastric cancer	CDH1	/	11	36	47
Endocrine neoplasia	MEN1	/	45	61	213
	RET	/	40	64	
	CDKN1B	/	3	0	
Von Hippel–Lindau syndrome	VHL	/	28	17	45
Hereditary paraganglioma–pheochromocytoma	SDH	/	66	98	184
	MAX	/	5	5	
	TMEM127	/	2	6	
	EPAS1	/	2	0	
Familial pituitary adenomas	AIP	/	10	4	14
Ataxia–telangiectasia	ATM	BI	23	5	59
		MONO	2	27	
	MRE11A	BI	0	0	
		MONO	0	2	
Hereditary papillary renal carcinoma	FH	/	20	12	37
	MET	/	3	2	
Hematologic malignancies	**	/	14	1	15
Hyperparathyroidism	CDC73	/	19	16	51

<table>
<tr><th>Predispositions</th><th>Genes</th><th>AR</th><th>IC+</th><th>REL+</th><th>Total</th></tr>
<tr><td rowspan="3">Cowden syndrome</td><td>CASR</td><td>/</td><td>16</td><td>0</td><td></td></tr>
<tr><td>PTEN</td><td>/</td><td>24</td><td>21</td><td rowspan="2">51</td></tr>
<tr><td>PIK3CA</td><td>/</td><td>6</td><td>0</td></tr>
<tr><td rowspan="4">Fanconi syndrome</td><td rowspan="2">FANC</td><td>BI</td><td>17</td><td>10</td><td rowspan="4">50</td></tr>
<tr><td>MONO</td><td>5</td><td>17</td></tr>
<tr><td rowspan="2">RAD51</td><td>BI</td><td>0</td><td>0</td></tr>
<tr><td>MONO</td><td>0</td><td>1</td></tr>
<tr><td rowspan="5">Familial malignant melanoma</td><td>CDKN2A</td><td>/</td><td>28</td><td>26</td><td rowspan="5">120</td></tr>
<tr><td>BAP1</td><td>/</td><td>31</td><td>11</td></tr>
<tr><td>MITF</td><td>/</td><td>20</td><td>0</td></tr>
<tr><td>POT1</td><td>/</td><td>3</td><td>0</td></tr>
<tr><td>CDK4</td><td>/</td><td>1</td><td>0</td></tr>
<tr><td rowspan="6">Neurofibromatosis</td><td>NF1</td><td>/</td><td>430</td><td>137</td><td rowspan="6">682</td></tr>
<tr><td>NF2</td><td>/</td><td>36</td><td>3</td></tr>
<tr><td>LZTR1</td><td>/</td><td>30</td><td>3</td></tr>
<tr><td>SMARCB1</td><td>/</td><td>10</td><td>3</td></tr>
<tr><td>SPRED1</td><td>/</td><td>18</td><td>8</td></tr>
<tr><td>SMARCE1</td><td>/</td><td>4</td><td>0</td></tr>
<tr><td>RASopathies and Noonan syndrome</td><td>***</td><td>/</td><td>159</td><td>NR</td><td>159</td></tr>
<tr><td>Retinoblastoma</td><td>RB1</td><td>/</td><td>29</td><td>6</td><td>35</td></tr>
<tr><td>Birt–Hogg–Dubé syndrome</td><td>FLCN</td><td>/</td><td>112</td><td>55</td><td>167</td></tr>
<tr><td rowspan="2">Bloom syndrome</td><td rowspan="2">BLM</td><td>BI</td><td>0</td><td>2</td><td rowspan="2">5</td></tr>
<tr><td>MONO</td><td>0</td><td>3</td></tr>
<tr><td rowspan="2">Carney complex</td><td>ARMC5</td><td>/</td><td>10</td><td>5</td><td rowspan="2">18</td></tr>
<tr><td>PRKAR1A</td><td>/</td><td>1</td><td>2</td></tr>
</table>

Predispositions	Genes	AR	IC+	REL+	Total
Gorlin syndrome	PTCH1	/	101	17	120
	PTCH2	/	1	0	
	SUFU	/	1	0	
Li–Fraumeni syndrome	TP53	/	31	39	71
	CHEK2	/	1	0	
Peutz–Jeghers syndrome	STK11	/	12	9	21
Juvenile polyposis syndrome	BMPR1A	/	7	9	36
	SMAD4	/	11	9	
Werner syndrome	WRN	BI	1	0	3
		MONO	0	2	
Xeroderma pigmentosum	XP	BI	11	15	43
		MONO	3	14	

Table I.1. *Statistics on index patients and their relatives carrying a genetic alteration predisposing to cancer, identified in in 2016 by the various accredited centers in France*

COMMENT ON TABLE I.1.– *Genes: names of the genes directly linked to the predisposition mentioned and which were reported in a diagnostic report, in France, in 2016. IC+: Index cases identified in 2016 as carriers of a genetic alteration in the genes mentioned; REL+: relatives identified in 2016 as carriers of a genetic alteration in the genes mentioned; AR: allelic status for genes with autosomal recessive transmission; BI: index or relatives carrying biallelic mutations; MONO: index or relatives carrying a monoallelic mutation; *constitutional hypermethylation of the promoter of the MLH1 gene; **CEBPA, ETV6, GATA2, KIT, MPL, SBDS, SH2B3, SRP72, WAS, etc.; ***BRAF, CBL, HRAS, KRAS, MAP2K1, MAP2K2, NRAS, PTPN11, RAF1, RIT1, SHOC2, SOS1, SOS2, etc.*

DEFINITION.– DNA methylation *is the enzymatically controlled addition of a methyl group to a nucleotide base (such as cytosine in eukaryotes) in a DNA molecule that plays a role in the regulation of gene expression (e.g., by inhibiting gene transcription).*

Genetic predisposition to cancer	*IC+ and REL+	%	Rank
Breast ovarian syndrome (including isolated ovarian cancers)	4,356	52.62	1
Lynch syndrome	1,148	13.87	2
Neurofibromatosis	682	8.24	3
Familial adenomatous polyposis	528	6.38	4
Endocrine neoplasia	213	2.57	5
Hereditary paraganglioma–pheochromocytoma	184	2.22	6
Birt–Hogg–Dubé syndrome	167	2.02	7
RASopathies and Noonan syndrome	159	1.92	8
Familial malignant melanoma	120	1.45	9
Gorlin syndrome	120	1.45	10
Li–Fraumeni syndrome	71	0.86	11
Ataxia–telangiectasia	59	0.71	12
Hyperparathyroidism	51	0.62	13
Cowden syndrome	51	0.62	14
Fanconi syndrome	50	0.60	15
Hereditary diffuse gastric cancer	47	0.57	16
von Hippel–Lindau syndrome	45	0.54	17
Xeroderma pigmentosum	43	0.52	18
Hereditary papillary renal carcinoma	37	0.45	19
Juvenile polyposis syndrome	36	0.43	20
Retinoblastoma	35	0.42	21
Peutz–Jeghers syndrome	21	0.25	22
Carney complex	18	0.22	23
Hematologic malignancies	15	0.18	24
Familial pituitary adenomas	14	0.17	25
Bloom syndrome	5	0.06	26
Werner syndrome	3	0.04	27
Total	8,278	100	/

Table I.2. *Order of syndromes according to their frequency (as deduced from statistics on index patients and their relatives carrying a genetic alteration predisposing to cancer, identified in the various accredited centers in France in 2016). *IC+ and REL+: index patient and relatives*

DEFINITION.– *Hematologic* malignancies *are hematologic cancers: cancers that occur in hematopoietic tissues, such as bone marrow, or in cells of the immune system. Leukemia, lymphoma, and multiple myeloma are examples of hematological cancers, also called* blood cancer.

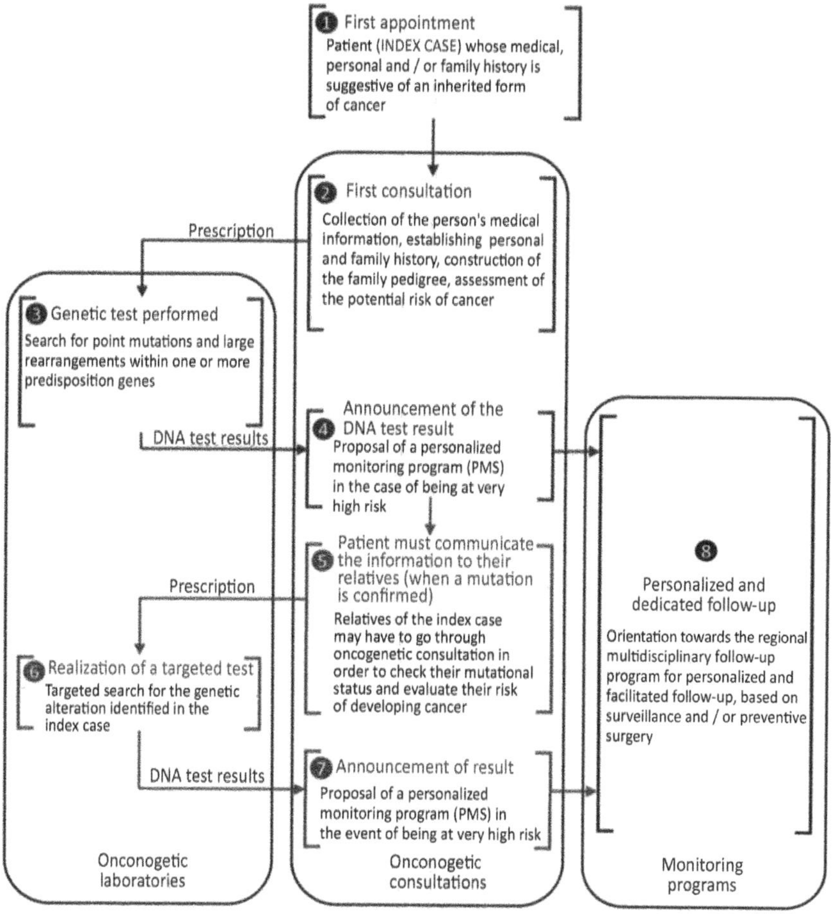

Figure I.1. *Global path of the index patient and their family members in the oncogenetic circuit in France*

PART 1

Major Syndromes

1

Hereditary Breast and Ovarian Cancer Syndrome Including Isolated Ovarian Cancers

In this chapter, we will describe the genetic predisposition to breast and ovarian cancers, including situations where the only cancers encountered are ovarian cancers.

1.1. Introduction

Inherited cancer syndromes are characterized by germline genetic mutations, which are associated with a high risk of cancer development. These mutations are usually inherited in an autosomal dominant manner and often induce cancers at a relatively early age. Hereditary cancer syndromes are rare, accounting for only about 5–10% of all breast cancers.

In addition to hereditary breast and ovarian cancer (HBOC, BRCA1/BRCA2) syndrome, breast and ovarian cancers are components of several autosomal dominant cancer syndromes: *Li–Fraumeni syndrome* (TP53), *Cowden syndrome* (PTEN) and *hereditary diffuse gastric cancer syndrome* (CDH1). The risk of breast cancer is higher in people diagnosed with these syndromes and there is a risk of developing tumors in other organs.

Other genetic syndromes may include breast cancer as an associated trait: the heterozygous carriers of the deleterious mutations of the ATM gene (*ataxia-telangiectasia*) and the STK11 gene (*Peutz–Jeghers syndrome*).

Lynch syndrome (LS) is primarily associated with colorectal and endometrial cancer, although several studies have shown that patients with LS have a higher risk of developing breast cancer.

Ovarian cancer is also associated with LS and *Gorlin syndrome*.

Mutations in other genes are also associated with an increased risk of developing breast cancer (checkpoint kinase 2 [CHEK2], PALB2, NBN and BARD1) or ovarian cancer (BRCA1 interacting protein 1 [BRIP1], RAD51C and RAD51D).

Recent studies have shown that half of the pathogenic mutations identified in individuals who meet only the HBOC test criteria were in genes other than BRCA1/2. Similarly, half of the pathogenic mutations identified in individuals who meet only the criteria for LS testing were in genes that are not part of the LS predisposition genes.

These same studies have shown the usefulness of testing people suspected of developing or who have developed HBOC for a list of 25 genes (BRCA1, BRCA2, ATM, CHEK2, PALB2, NBN, BARD1, BRIP1, RAD51C, RAD51D, MLH1, MSH2, EPCAM, MSH6, PMS2, APC, MUTYH (biallelic), BMPR1A, SMAD4, TP53, PTEN, STK11, CDH1, CDKN2A and CDK4).

While MUTYH biallelic mutations are known to cause *MYH polyposis-associated syndrome* with a 28-fold increased risk of colorectal adenocarcinoma, monoallelic carriers have been reported to have only a slight increase in colorectal cancer risk (odds ratio of ~1.34), but together with an increased risk of breast cancer.

The most recent studies have confirmed the association of 15 genes with an increased risk (>2.0 times) of breast cancer (ATM, BARD1, BRCA1, BRCA2, CDH1, CDKN2A, CHEK2 (except p.I157T), MLH1, MSH2, MSH6, NF1, PALB2, PTEN, RAD51D and TP53). Eleven genes were associated with an increased risk (>2.0 times) of ovarian cancer (ATM, BRCA1, BRCA2, BRIP1, MSH2, MSH6, NBN, PMS2, RAD51C, RAD51D and TP53).

In this section, we will discuss the roles of BRCA1 and BRCA2 genes in predisposition to both breast and ovarian cancers; CHEK2, PALB2, NBN and BARD1 in predisposition to breast cancer; and BRIP1, RAD51C and RAD51D in predisposition to ovarian cancer.

1.2. Prevalence

Approximately one in 300–400 people in the general population is born with an inherited mutation in the BRCA1 or BRCA2 gene. The frequency of BRCA1 or BRCA2 mutation is approximately one in 40 in the Ashkenazi Jewish population.

PALB2 pathogenic variants have been examined in multiple small studies of familial and early breast cancer in multiple populations. The prevalence of pathogenic variants ranged from 0.4% to 3.9%. Similar to BRIP1 and CHEK2, there was incomplete segregation of PALB2 pathogenic variants in families with hereditary breast cancer.

It is estimated that mutations in RAD51C increase the risk of ovarian cancer by 9% and occur in approximately 1–5.7% of women with ovarian cancer (without considering any selection criteria).

It is estimated that one in 200 people with ovarian cancer will have a constitutional mutation in the RAD51D gene.

When should one suspect a genetic predisposition? The following section outlines the criteria for referral for an oncogenetic consultation, according to the National Comprehensive Cancer Network (NCCN).

1.2.1. *Genetic risk assessment criteria*[1]

1.2.1.1. *A person with cancer*

For a diagnosed patient, the reasons for referral for an oncogenetic consultation, according to the NCCN, are as follows:

1) a person with ovarian cancer[2];

2) a person diagnosed with breast cancer who meets one of the following criteria:

– a mutation known in the family in a cancer predisposition gene,

– diagnosed with breast cancer at an age ≤ 50 years,

1 The criteria for risk assessment and genetic testing are not identical. For the purposes of these guidelines, invasive breast cancer and ductal carcinoma *in situ* should be included. The maternal and paternal sides of the family should be considered independently for familial forms of cancer.

2 This includes fallopian tubes and primary peritoneal cancers. BRCA-related ovarian cancers are associated with non-mucinous epithelial histology. Lynch syndrome may be associated with both non-mucinous and mucinous epithelial tumors. Clinical signs of Lynch syndrome should be monitored. Specific types of non-epithelial ovarian cancers and tumors may also be associated with other rare syndromes. Examples include an association between tumors of the sex cord with annular tubules and Peutz–Jeghers syndrome or Sertoli–Leydig tumors and DICER-related disorders.

– a triple negative breast cancer (ER^-, PR^-, $HER2^-$) diagnosed at an age ≤ 60 years,

– two primary[3] breast cancers in a single individual,

– breast cancer at any age,

– one or more relatives with breast cancer at an age ≤ 50 years,

– one or more relatives with invasive ovarian cancer at any age,

– two or more relatives[4] with breast cancer, prostate cancer (Gleason score > 7 or metastatic) and/or pancreatic cancer at any age,

– personal history of pancreatic cancer at any age,

– belonging to a population at increased risk[5],

– male breast cancer;

3) an individual with metastatic prostate cancer (radiographic evidence or disease confirmed by biopsy);

4) a person of Ashkenazi Jewish descent with breast, ovarian or pancreatic cancer at any age;

5) a person with a personal history of one of the following and/or three or more affected family members (especially if diagnosed at ≤ 50 years of age and may include several primary cancers in one person): breast cancer, pancreatic cancer, prostate cancer (Gleason score > 7 or metastatic), melanoma, sarcoma, adrenal cortical carcinoma, brain tumors, leukemia, diffuse gastric cancer[6], colon cancer, endometrial cancer, thyroid cancer, kidney cancer, dermatological manifestations[7] and/or macrocephaly, or hamartomatous polyps of the gastrointestinal tract[8].

---

3 Two primary breast cancers include bilateral (contralateral) neoplasia or two (or more) distinct homolateral primary tumors diagnosed either synchronously or asynchronously.

4 Close blood relatives include first-, second-, and third-degree relatives.

5 For populations at increased risk due to founding mutations, inclusion requirements may be modified.

6 For lobular breast cancer with a family history of diffuse gastric cancer, CDH1 gene testing should be considered.

7 For dermatological manifestations, see section 14.1.1 for Cowden syndrome.

8 For hamartomatous colon polyps in association with breast cancer and hyperpigmented macules of the lips and oral mucosa, an STK11 test should be considered (Peutz–Jeghers syndrome). Melanomas have been reported in some BRCA-related families.

DEFINITION.– Macrocephaly *refers to an oversized head in infants. It is not a condition in itself, but may be a symptom of other conditions or complications. Macrocephaly is defined as head circumference greater than two standard deviations (SD) above the mean value for a given age and sex.*

DEFINITION.– *A* polyp *is a growth protruding from a mucous membrane.*

1.2.1.2. *Person with no personal history of cancer*

An individual with no personal history of cancer, but with:

1) a close relative with one of the following:

i) a mutation known in the family affecting a cancer predisposition gene,

ii) two or more primary breast cancers in the same individual,

iii) two or more individuals with primary breast cancers belonging to the same family branch with at least one diagnosed at an age ≤ 50 years,

iv) ovarian cancer,

v) male breast cancer;

2) a first- or second-degree relative with breast cancer at an age ≤ 45;

3) a family history of three cases or more of the following (especially if diagnosed at ≤ 50 years of age; may include several primary cancers in the same individual): breast cancer, pancreatic cancer, prostate cancer (Gleason score ≥ 7 or metastatic), melanoma, sarcoma, adrenal cortical carcinoma, brain tumors, leukemia, diffuse gastric cancer, colorectal cancer, endometrial cancer, thyroid cancer, kidney cancer, dermatologic manifestations, and/or macrocephaly, or hamartomatous polyps of the gastrointestinal tract.

DEFINITION.– Melanoma *is a form of cancer that begins in melanocytes (cells that make the pigment melanin). It can start in a mole (skin melanoma), but can also start in other pigmented tissues, such as the eye or intestines.*

DEFINITION.– *The term* sarcoma *generally refers to a broad group of cancers that begin in bone and soft tissue (also called* connective *tissue) (soft tissue sarcoma). Soft tissue sarcoma forms in the tissues that connect, support and surround other body structures. This includes muscle, fat, blood vessels, nerves, tendons and the lining of joints.*

1.3. Indications for genetic testing

The NCCN also now recognizes that multigene panel testing for hereditary forms of cancer can be more efficient and cost effective. It has been shown that 7% of patients with a previously uninformative genetic test had a pathogenic mutation with a multigene panel test.

As such, a thorough family history should not be limited to breast cancer and should include the identification of cancers of other organs that may be part of a breast cancer syndrome or other inherited cancer syndromes.

In patients whose personal or family history suggests more than one hereditary cancer syndrome, or in patients with such a history who have tested negative for a single gene, the NCCN suggests that multigene panel tests should be offered.

NOTE.– Inheriting a BRCA2 or PALB2 mutation from both parents causes specific types of Fanconi anemia. This rare condition is characterized by progressive bone marrow dysfunction, growth delay, variable birth defects, and a high risk of leukemia and early onset solid tumors.

A male or female with a confirmed BRCA2 or PALB2 mutation may therefore consider preconception genetic counseling to clarify the risks in case their partner also carries a mutation in the same gene.

Several organizations have recommended that the BRCA1/2 germline mutation test be offered to all women with epithelial ovarian, tubal or peritoneal cancer, regardless of their histotype, age or family history.

1.4. Tumors

1.4.1. *Breast*

In terms of histologic types, most breast cancers associated with BRCA1 are of no special type (NST), involving invasive ductal adenocarcinoma and having higher grade than sporadic breast cancers. In terms of molecular subtypes, the majority of BRCA1 breast cancers can therefore be classified as basal-like.

DEFINITION.– Adenocarcinoma *is a tumor that begins in glandular (secretory) cells. Glandular cells are found in the tissues that line certain internal organs and produce and release substances in the body, such as mucus, digestive juices, or other fluids. Most of the cancers in the breast, pancreas, lung, prostate and colon are adenocarcinomas.*

Like BRCA1-associated tumors and sporadic carcinomas, BRCA2-associated breast cancers are predominantly NST invasive ductal adenocarcinomas with moderate to poor differentiation. However, the overexpression of the estrogen receptor, progesterone receptor, CK8 and CK18 allow BRCA2 tumors to be classified in the luminal molecular subtype, with the vast majority belonging to luminal subtype B.

Most BRCA1 carcinomas have a basal phenotype and are high grade, highly proliferative, estrogen receptor negative and HER2 negative mammary carcinomas characterized by the expression of basal markers such as basal keratins, P-cadherin and epidermal growth factor receptor (EGFR). BRCA1 carcinomas frequently carry p53 mutations. The basal-type phenotype is only occasionally encountered in BRCA2 carcinomas, which tend to be estrogen and progesterone receptor positive. Loss of heterozygosity of BRCA1 and BRCA2 is found in almost all BRCA1 and BRCA2 carcinomas, respectively. Both genotypes have a low frequency of HER2 overexpression/amplification. Other reports suggest that BRCA2-related tumors include excess lobular and tubulo-lobular histology.

In summary, the histological characteristics associated with the pathogenic variants of BRCA2 have been inconsistent.

Concerning the histological subtype, no correlation has been found with the most frequent germline variant in northern Europe, 1100delC of CHEK2. However, it has been shown that in Poland, where there are two other founder variants with a higher prevalence than 1100delC, the I157T mutation is associated with the lobular carcinoma subtype.

An examination of pathological features in 10 families with pathogenic RAD51C mutations revealed that nine patients (47%) developed carcinomas of the ovary and 12 (63%) developed carcinomas of the breast. This review also noted that, as a group, the RAD51C-associated mammary carcinomas were diagnosed at an early stage (89%) and were hormone receptor positive, HER2 negative, moderately differentiated invasive ductal carcinomas (IDC) and NST (80%).

In addition, RAD51C breast carcinomas were comparable to BRCA2-associated breast carcinomas in their lack of specific pathologic features and their tendency to be ER positive and HER2 negative, differing only in the Ki-67 proliferation index, which is significantly higher in BRCA2 tumors.

1.4.2. *Ovaries*

In terms of gynecological cancers, women with BRCA1 mutations have a 50% risk of developing ovarian, tubal or peritoneal carcinoma, while in BRCA2 carriers, the risk is about 25% for all ovarian cancer patients and about a quarter of patients with high-grade serous carcinoma (HGSC).

Carriers of BRCA mutations do not appear to have an increased risk of developing endometrial cancer, although there is some evidence to suggest that there may be an increased risk for serous/serous-like endometrial cancer.

BRCA1/2 carriers develop tumors that are almost always of high-grade serous histology, but the tumors may also be endometrioid and, more rarely, have clear cell histology.

Currently, there is a strong belief that the BRCA1/2 syndrome is almost exclusively associated with the histotype of ovarian cancer: HGSC.

Primary site histological features that have been found to be more common in HGSCs associated with BRCA1 (germinal or somatic) mutations include a solid, pseudo-endometrioid, transitional appearance (SET) , increased numbers of tumor infiltrating lymphocytes (TIL), and higher mitotic index and necrosis.

BRCA2 mutations have also been associated with an increased risk of developing pancreatic and prostate cancer.

Cancer sites	BRCA1		BRCA2	
	Weight of evidence	Absolute risk magnitude	Weight of evidence	Absolute risk magnitude
Breast (female)	+++	High	+++	High
Ovary, fallopian tubes, peritoneum	+++	High	+++	Moderate
Breast (male)	+	Not defined	+++	Low
Pancreas	++	Very low	+++	Low
Prostate	+	Not defined	+++	High

Table 1.1. *Spectrum of cancers in carriers of BRCA1 and BRCA2 pathogenic variants*

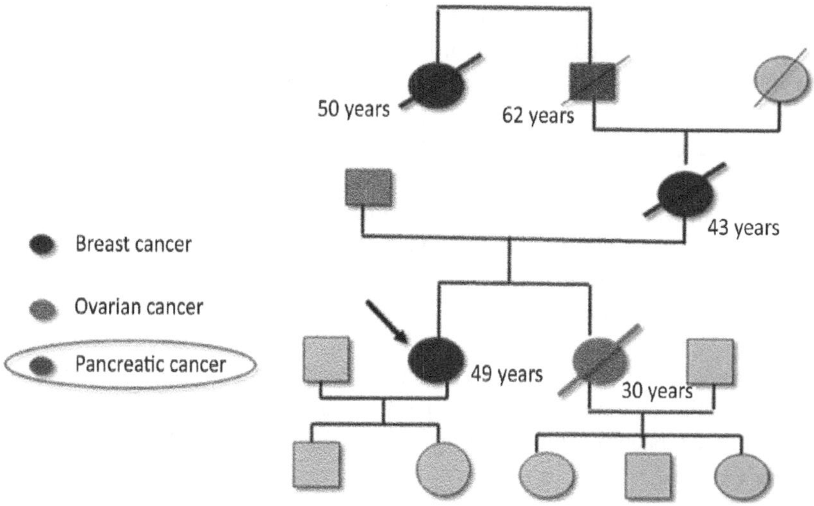

Figure 1.1. *Familial pancreatic cancer in a syndromic context; identification of a mutation in the BRCA2 gene in the index case (indicated by an arrow). For a color version of this figure, see www.iste.co.uk/boukhatem/oncogenetics.zip*

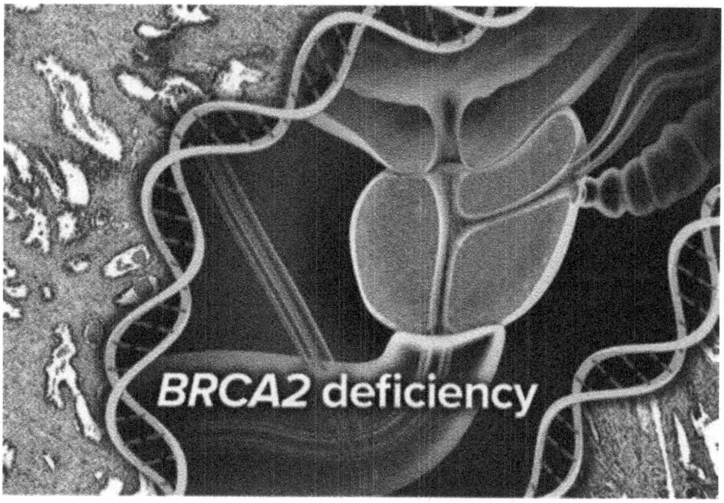

Figure 1.2. *BRCA2 mutations are associated with breast and ovarian cancer, but also increase the risk of prostate cancer in men*

Other genes in the BRCA1/2 pathway (repair of double-stranded DNA breaks) have also been implicated in hereditary ovarian cancer; in particular, mutations in RAD51C, RAD51D and BRIP1 confer ~10% increased risk of ovarian cancer.

Studies have identified RAD51C, RAD51D, BRIP1 and FANCM as likely susceptibility genes, particularly for the high-grade serous ovarian carcinoma (HGSOC) histotype (high-grade epithelial tumors of the serous and endometrioid subtypes). In a subset of 10 families carrying RAD51C deleterious mutations, ovarian carcinomas histotypes were as follows: (56%), low-grade serous carcinoma (LGSC) (11%), high-grade endometrioid (11%) and unclassified (22%).

Deleterious mutations in the gene are associated with a moderate increase in the risk of epithelial ovarian cancer (EOC). The relative risks associated with BRIP1 mutations have been estimated to be 11.22 for invasive EOC and 14.09 for high-grade serous.

1.5. Genes

1.5.1. *BRCA1*

The BRCA1 gene codes for a 220 kDa (1,863 amino acids) nuclear polypeptide. The BRCA1 protein has been implicated in various cellular processes, including repair of DNA damage and regulation of the transcription cycle, chromatin remodeling and ubiquitination. More recently, it has been shown to play a role in splicing and mediating estrogenic metabolites.

1.5.2. *BRCA2*

BRCA2 encodes a protein of 3418 amino acids and contains repeats of 39 amino acids that are critical for the binding of RAD51 recombinase (RAD51), a protein necessary for the repair of recombinant DNA. BRCA2 appears to have a more restricted role, largely limited to recombinant DNA repair and regulation of RAD51.

1.5.3. *CHEK2*

The CHEK2 gene codes for a cell cycle checkpoint regulatory protein and therefore this gene is a putative tumor suppressor. It contains an associated protein interaction domain at the fork head, essential for activation in response to DNA damage and is rapidly phosphorylated in response to replication blockages and DNA damage.

1.5.4. *PALB2*

The partner and localizer gene of BRCA2 (PALB2) encodes a protein that can function in tumor suppression. This protein binds and colocalizes with the BRCA2 protein in nuclear foci and likely allows stable intranuclear localization and accumulation of BRCA2.

1.5.5. *NBN*

The nibrin gene (NBN): mutations in this gene are associated with Nijmegen breakage syndrome, an autosomal recessive chromosomal instability syndrome characterized by microcephaly, growth delay, immunodeficiency and a predisposition to cancer. The coded protein is a member of the MRE11/RAD50 double-strand break repair that consists of five proteins. The protein is thought to be involved in the repair of double-stranded DNA breaks and in the activation of check points induced by DNA damage.

DEFINITION.– Microcephaly *is an abnormality of the head (small size), a congenital condition associated with incomplete brain development.*

1.5.6. *BARD1*

The BRCA1 gene associated RING domain 1 (BARD1) encodes a protein that interacts with the N-terminal region of BRCA1. In addition to its ability to bind BRCA1 *in vivo* and *in vitro*, it shares homology with the two most conserved regions of BRCA1: the N-terminal RING pattern and the C-terminal BRCT domain. The formation of a stable complex between the BRCA1/BARD1 proteins may be an essential aspect of the tumor suppressor function of BRCA1.

1.5.7. *BRIP1*

The BRIP1 gene codes for a protein member of the RecQ DEAH helicase family and interacts with the BRCT repeats of the protein encoded by BRCA1. The attachment complex is important for the normal double-strand breaks repair function of BRCA1.

1.5.8. *RAD51C*

RAD51C is a member of the RAD51 family and is an essential component of homologous recombination. It is localized on chromosome 17q23 and codes for strand transfer proteins.

1.5.9. *RAD51D*

RAD51D is another of the RAD51 paralogues and also codes for proteins involved in homologous recombinant repair of DNA damage.

1.6. Genotype–phenotype correlations

Some genotype–phenotype correlations have been identified in families carrying BRCA2 pathogenic variants.

In studies totaling 189 families with pathogenic variants of BRCA2, an ovarian cancer cluster region was identified in exon 11 between nucleotides 3035 and 6629.

Pathogenic variants in the ovarian cancer cluster region were associated with an increased risk of ovarian cancer and a decreased risk of breast cancer compared to families with variants on either side of this region.

In addition, a study confirmed by other studies involving 356 families with truncated protein pathogenic variants of BRCA1 showed that the risk of breast cancer was lower with variants from the central region (nucleotides 2401–4190). The risk of ovarian cancer was significantly reduced with variants in the 3' end region of the gene at nucleotide 4191.

Higher rates of ovarian cancer have been found in BRCA1:185delAG carriers at the 5' end of BRCA1 compared to BRCA1:5382insC carriers at the 3' end of the gene.

The risk of breast cancer, particularly bilateral breast cancer, and the occurrence of breast and ovarian cancer in the same individual appear to be higher in carriers of the pathogenic variant BRCA1:5382insC than in carriers of BRCA1:185delAG and BRCA2:6174delT. The risk of ovarian cancer is significantly higher in BRCA1 pathogenic variant carriers, and is rare before age 45 in BRCA2:6174delT carriers.

1.7. Penetrance

DEFINITION.– Penetrance *refers to the likelihood that a clinical condition will occur when a particular genotype is present. A condition is said to have incomplete penetrance when some individuals carrying the pathogenic variant express the associated trait while others do not. It is expressed as the percentage of cases that express the associated phenotype among all carriers of the pathogenic variant.*

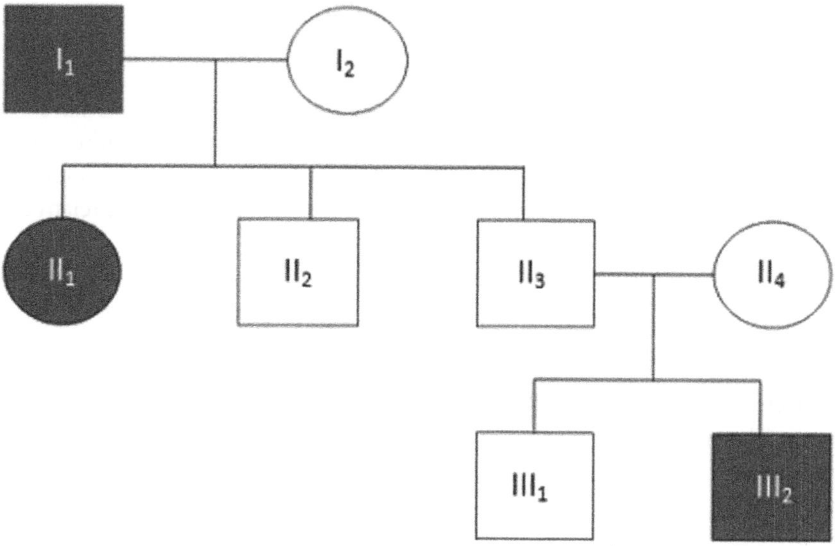

Figure 1.3. *Incomplete penetrance. Individual II3 is an obligatory carrier of the genetic anomaly (their father is sick, they have a sick sister and son as well), but they express a normal phenotype*

Carriers of deleterious BRCA1/2 mutations have a cumulative breast cancer risk of 50–85% and an ovarian cancer risk of 15–60% at age 70.

The increased risk of contralateral breast cancer (CBC) in carriers of pathogenic BRCA1 and BRCA2 variants has been confirmed in several large studies. Estimates of the 10-year cumulative risk of CBC in BRCA1/2 carriers range from 18% to 34% for BRCA1 pathogenic variants and 11% to 29% for BRCA2 pathogenic variants.

It is also estimated that the risk of bilateral breast cancer at age 60 is as high as 64% in carriers of BRCA1 mutations diagnosed with breast cancer.

CBC risk was also inversely correlated with age in some studies, with the highest risks observed in women whose first case of breast cancer occurred before the age of 40.

The risk of ovarian cancer is estimated to be 39% for carriers of pathogenic BRCA1 variants and 11–17% for carriers of pathogenic BRCA2 variants.

PALB2 mutations have been shown to confer an absolute breast cancer risk of 33–58% at age 70.

Mutations leading to the production of truncated CHEK2 proteins have been associated with a clinically significant risk of breast cancer in mutation carriers without an affected first- or second-degree relative (20%), and this risk may be as high as 44% in mutation carriers with an affected first- or second-degree relative.

The CHEK2 mutation associated with a family history of breast cancer results in a 28–37% lifetime risk of breast carcinoma, but does not increase the risk of ovarian cancer.

Inactivating variants of BRIP1 are associated with an increased risk of breast cancer. The monoallelic mutations in BRIP1 confer a relative risk of 2.0 for the development of breast cancer. However, there is incomplete segregation of the pathogenic variants BRIP1 and CHEK2 with breast cancer.

Although the data for RAD51C are conflicting, among these data there is substantial evidence of a modest association between germline variants of RAD51C and breast and ovarian cancers.

NOTE.– The genes widely recognized as conferring a risk of breast or ovarian cancer are distributed as follows:

– breast cancer: BRCA1, BRCA2, PALB2, PTEN, STK11, TP53;

– ovarian cancer: BRCA1, BRCA2, MLH1, MSH2, MSH6, PMS2, RAD51C, RAD51D.

For breast cancer:

– it has been agreed that ATM and CHEK2 confer a moderately increased risk of breast cancer, but concerns about the interpretation of the results of these genes led to a recommendation that only truncated variants be reported, in addition to ATM c.7217T > G (p. Val2424Gly), which is recognized as conferring an increased risk of breast cancer;

– CDH1 has also been shown to confer a risk of breast cancer, but only in the specific case of lobular breast cancer;

– insufficient evidence has been found for a significant risk of breast cancer associated with NBN, BRIP1 or BARD1.

For ovarian cancer, it has been accepted that BRIP1 confers a sufficient risk of ovarian cancer, so a prophylactic bilateral adnexectomy should be considered.

1.8. Mode of transmission

These predispositions are usually inherited in an autosomal dominant mode and are often characterized by early onset of disease.

1.9. Risks to family members: special consideration

Inheriting BRCA2 or PALB2 mutations from both parents causes specific types of Fanconi anemia. This rare condition is characterized by progressive bone marrow dysfunction, growth delay, variable congenital malformations, a high risk of leukemia and early solid tumors.

A woman and man with a confirmed BRCA2 or PALB2 mutation may therefore consider preconception genetic counseling to clarify the risks their partner has of also carrying a mutation in the same gene.

Current guidelines emphasize the importance of recognizing pancreatic cancer and the risk of prostate cancer associated with BRCA1/2 mutations. The risk of developing pancreatic cancer has been shown to be two to three times higher in patients with BRCA1 mutations and two to seven times higher in patients with BRCA2 mutations, respectively.

1.10. Monitoring

The surveillance recommendations for carriers of deleterious BRCA1/2 mutations according to the NCCN are as follows.

1.10.1. *Women*

There should be a breast awareness program[9] from the age of 18. Clinical examination of the breasts should take place every 6–12 months[10] from the age of 25 years and should include:

– breast monitoring[11]:

- 25–29 years of age: annual breast cancer screening with contrast MRI[12,13] (or mammography with consideration of tomosynthesis, only if MRI is not available) or individualized screening based on family history if breast cancer is diagnosed before the age of 30,

- between 30 and 75 years of age: annual mammography taking into account tomosynthesis and breast MRI screening with contrast,

- over 75 years of age: monitoring should be considered on an individual basis,

- for women with a BRCA1/2 mutation who are being treated for breast cancer and have not undergone bilateral mastectomy, screening by annual mammography and breast MRI should continue as described above;

---

9 Women should know their breasts and promptly report changes to their treating physicians. Periodic breast self-examination can help to recognize breast changes. In premenopausal women, the most informative self-examinations are those performed at the end of menstruation.

10 Randomized trials comparing the performance of clinical breast examination to its absence have not been conducted. The rationale for recommending a clinical breast examination every 6–12 months stems from the concern that breast cancer may develop in the time between examinations.

11 The suitability of imaging modalities and their programming are still under investigation.

12 Breast MRI is preferred because of the theoretical risk of radiation exposure in mutation carriers.

13 Limitations of high-quality breast MRI include the need for a dedicated breast coil, the ability to perform an MRI-guided biopsy, experienced breast MRI radiologists and regional availability. Breast MRI is preferably performed on days 7–15 of the menstrual cycle in premenopausal women.

– discussing the option of risk-reducing mastectomy: the counseling should include a discussion of the degree of protection, reconstruction options and risks. In addition, family history and residual risk of breast cancer with age and life expectancy should be considered during counseling;

– recommending risk reduction by offering prophylactic[14] bilateral adnexectomy (PBA), usually between 35 and 40 years of age and at the end of maternity. For the management of ovarian cancer risk in patients with BRCA2 mutations, it is reasonable to delay PBA until 40-45 years of age (ovarian cancer development in patients with BRCA2 mutations is on average 8-10 years later than in patients with BRCA1 mutations):

- guidance includes a discussion of reproductive desires, the extent of cancer risk, the degree of protection against breast and ovarian cancer, management of menopausal symptoms, possible short-term hormone replacement therapy and related medical issues,

- bilateral adnexectomy alone is not the standard of care for risk reduction, although clinical trials of bilateral prophylactic interval adnexectomy and delayed oophorectomy are ongoing. The only concern with bilateral adnexectomy is that women are still at risk of developing ovarian cancer. In addition, in premenopausal women, oophorectomy probably reduces the risk of developing breast cancer, but the extent of this reduction is uncertain and depends on gene alteration;

– addressing the psychosocial, social and quality of life aspects of prophylactic bilateral mastectomy and adnexectomy.

For patients who have not chosen PBA, transvaginal ultrasound combined with serum CA-125 for ovarian cancer screening, although of uncertain benefit, may be considered from 30 to 35 years of age.

Appropriate medication (e.g. tamoxifen, raloxifene, anastrozole and exemestane) can almost halve the risk of developing hormone-positive breast cancer. The decision to use such a drug requires discussion of the relative benefits and potential risk of side effects in the context of a woman's general health, menopausal status and reproductive plans. In addition, the use of PARP inhibitors (e.g. olaparib, niraparib and rucaparib) is a potentially lethal synthetic therapeutic strategy and can be considered as targeted chemoprevention in patients with specific defects in DNA repair including BRCA1/2 mutations.

14 In view of the high rate of occult neoplasia, particular attention should be paid to the sampling and pathological examination of the ovaries and fallopian tubes.

DEFINITION.– *The term* mastectomy *refers to the surgical removal of all or part of the breast and sometimes the associated lymph nodes and muscles.*

DEFINITION.– *The term* bilateral adnexectomy *refers to a surgical procedure that involves the removal of the fallopian tubes and ovaries on both sides of the reproductive organ.*

DEFINITION.– *The term* prophylactic *here refers to a medical act that tends to prevent or inhibit the spread or occurrence of a cancerous disease.*

1.10.2. *Men*[15]

It is recommended to practice breast self-examination from the age of 35.

A clinical breast examination is recommended every 12 months from the age of 35 onwards.

From the age of 45, the recommendations are as follows:

– recommended prostate cancer screening for BRCA2 carriers;

– considered screening for prostate cancer in BRCA1 carriers.

1.10.3. *Men and women*

People at risk need to be educated to recognize the signs and symptoms of cancer, particularly those associated with BRCA1/2 mutations.

There are no specific guidelines for screening for pancreatic cancer and melanoma, but screening can be individualized according to the cancer types observed in the family[16].

1.10.4. *Risks to relatives*

Relatives should be advised about the possible risks of hereditary cancer, options for risk assessment and management.

---

15 There are limited data to support breast imaging in men.

16 Whole skin and eye examinations are required for melanomas and investigation protocols for pancreatic cancer.

It is necessary to recommend genetic counseling and to consider genetic testing for at-risk relatives.

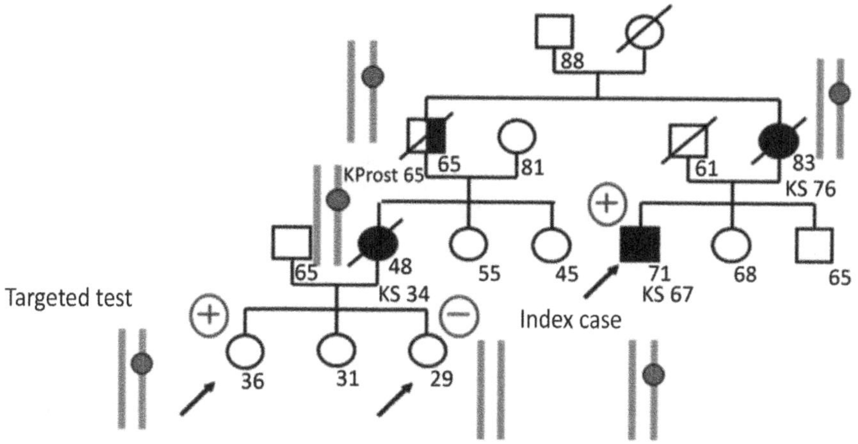

Figure 1.4. *Identifying at-risk individuals in the family (by testing family members (adults) who wish to be tested to reassure non-carriers and monitor carriers). The targeted test in the 36-year-old female was positive and the test in the 29-year-old female was negative*

1.10.5. *Reproductive options*

For patients of childbearing age, it is recommended to advise them on options for prenatal diagnosis and assisted human reproduction, including preimplantation genetic diagnosis. The discussion should include the known risks, limitations and benefits of these technologies.

Biallelic mutations in some genes, such as BRCA2 and some other genes included in gene panels, may be associated with rare autosomal recessive conditions. Thus, for these types of genes, partner testing for mutations in the same gene would be considered if it were to be used as a basis for reproductive decision making and/or risk assessment and management.

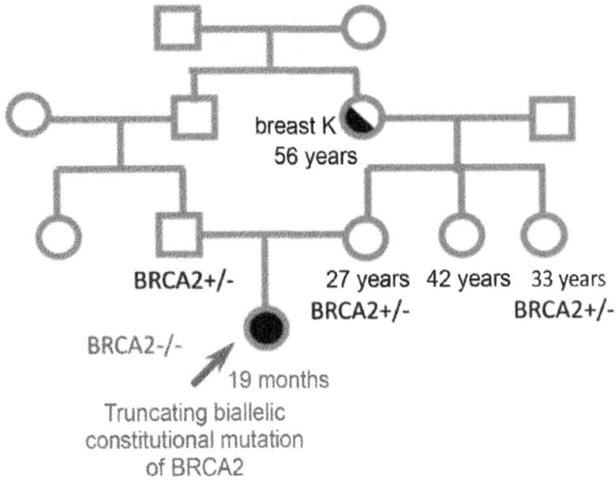

Figure 1.5. *Fanconi disease: autosomal recessive transmission. Both parents are carriers of BRCA2 mutations. Medical history of the baby includes abnormalities of fetal development, small size, bone marrow dysplasia, Wilms' tumor at 7 months, neuroblastoma at 11 months and medulloblastoma tumor at 19 months*

DEFINITION.– Medulloblastoma *is a rapidly growing type of cancer that forms in the cerebellum. Medulloblastoma tends to spread through cerebrospinal fluid to the spinal cord or other parts of the brain. It can also spread to other parts of the body, but this is rare. Medulloblastoma is more common in children and young adults. It is a type of embryonic tumor of the central nervous system.*

DEFINITION.– Neuroblastoma *is a type of cancer that develops from immature nerve cells. It usually begins in the adrenal glands, but can also start in the abdomen, chest or nerve-vessel tissues near the spine. Neuroblastoma occurs most often in children under 5 years of age. It is thought to begin before birth.*

DEFINITION.– Wilms' tumor *is a rare kidney cancer that mainly affects children. Also known as nephroblastoma, it is the most common kidney cancer in children. Wilms' tumor most often affects children between the ages of 3 and 4 years and becomes much less common after the age of 5 years.*

Currently, it is generally recommended that women with PALB2 mutations follow the breast cancer risk management guidelines described above for women with BRCA1/2 mutations.

Carriers of CHEK2 and NBN mutations are also eligible for breast MRI screening since their cumulative lifetime risk is greater than 20%. The magnitude of the lifetime risk associated with some low penetrance genes is unclear, such as RAD51C and BARD1, and as such, MRI is not recommended in these cases.

The NCCN guidelines currently suggest active breast MRI monitoring for patients with CHEK constitutional mutations.

For patients with deleterious RAD51C mutations, NCCN recommends prophylactic bilateral adnexectomy to reduce risk but states that routine monitoring or intervention for breast cancer is not indicated due to insufficient evidence.

It has been accepted that BRIP1 confers a sufficient risk of ovarian cancer, so prophylactic bilateral adnexectomy should be considered.

2

Lynch Syndrome

2.1. Introduction

Lynch syndrome (LS) is the most common form of hereditary colorectal cancer (CRC), and previously it was called hereditary non-polyposis colorectal cancer (HNPCC).

LS is an inherited tumor predisposing condition caused by mutations in the DNA mismatch repair (MMR) genes (MLH1, MSH2, MSH6 or PMS2) or in the EPCAM gene, which inactivates MSH2 via promoter hypermethylation.

Cancers associated with LS are characterized by a high degree of microsatellite instability (MSI-H) resulting from the defect in the MMR pathway (MMR-D) and high rates of DNA mutations, particularly in microsatellites.

DEFINITION.– Microsatellite instability (MSI) *refers to a characteristic of cells that contain an abnormality in DNA MMR. For example, the presence of MSI in colorectal tumor tissue can be used as a marker for germline mutations in one of the DNA MMR genes associated with LS. The MSI phenotype can also occur sporadically and in these cases is linked to gene hypermethylation. This is a problem in the differential diagnosis of LS.*

In addition to colorectal cancer and endometrial cancer (EC), which are the most common, LS is also associated with other gastrointestinal cancers and non-gastrointestinal malignancies, including those of the genitourinary tract.

It has been shown that the ovary, stomach, hepatobiliary tract, small intestine, brain and skin cancers develop with increased incidence in LS, while increased incidence in breast cancer, prostate cancer, pancreatic cancer (PC) and sarcomas remain uncertain.

Constitutional Oncogenetics,

Recent data indicate that two of the LS predisposing genes, MSH6 and PMS2, are associated with an increased risk of breast cancer.

The association of LS with urothelial cancers is relatively new. Urothelial cancers have only recently been included in the criteria that aid in the diagnosis of LS. In addition, an increased risk of bladder cancer in patients with LS has been reported. These cancers may result from the downstream presence of primary upper tract cancers and may not represent primary bladder cancers.

The cumulative risk of PC in LS patients is approximately 3.7% (1.5% in the general population).

Two variants of the disease are recognized. Muir–Torre syndrome (MTS) has been recognized as a distinct variant of LS, with more than 200 cases reported worldwide. MTS is typically characterized by at least one visceral malignancy and skin neoplasia.

Another subtype of LS is Turcot syndrome (TS) (co-occurrence of a brain tumor with a colorectal tumor in the same individual), phenotypically distinct from MTS, which typically presents brain gliomas/glioblastomas.

DEFINITION.– Glioblastoma *is a type of fast-growing tumor of the central nervous system that forms from the glial (supporting) tissues of the brain and spinal cord and whose cells are very different from normal cells. Glioblastoma usually occurs in adults and affects the brain more often than the spinal cord, also known as glioblastoma multiform and grade IV astrocytoma.*

TS can be dominant or recessive. The dominant TS form is due to heterozygous mutations in the MMR genes or in the adenomatous polyposis (APC) gene. The recessive TS form is due to a biallelic mutation in the MMR genes and can also be classified as constitutional mismatch repair deficiency (CMMR-D) syndrome (but not vice versa: only a minority of CMMR-D cases meet the diagnostic criteria for TS). The predominant brain tumor in APC-associated TS is medulloblastoma, while glioblastoma predominates in TS associated with mutations in the MMR genes.

It should be noted that tumors generally develop in carriers of biallelic MMR mutations at a very young age: hematological malignancies usually occur in childhood or early childhood (mean age of onset: 5.5 years), whereas brain tumors develop somewhat later in childhood (mean age: 8 years).

Syndrome	Predisposition gene	Mode of transmission	Characteristic type of brain tumor
Turcot	APC	AD	Medulloblastoma
	MSH2, MLH1, MSH6, PMS2	AD or AR	Glioblastoma
CMMR-D constitutional MMR deficiencies	MSH2, MLH1, MSH6, PMS2	AR	Astrocytoma

Table 2.1. *Subtypes of Lynch syndrome (AD: autosomal dominant; AR: autosomal recessive)*

2.2. Prevalence

A recent study using a large dataset from familial colon cancer registries produced new estimates of the prevalence of high-risk mutations in key CRC susceptibility genes: it was estimated that 1/279 (95% IC, 1/192–1/403) of the population carries mutations in one of the MMR genes (MLH1 = 1/1,946, MSH2 = 1/2,841, MSH6 = 1/758, PMS2 = 1/714), and 1/45 carries mutations in MUTYH (monoallelic).

LS accounts for 2–4% of all CRC cases and about 2.5% of EC cases. In fact, one in 35 CRCs and one in 50 ECs are attributable to LS.

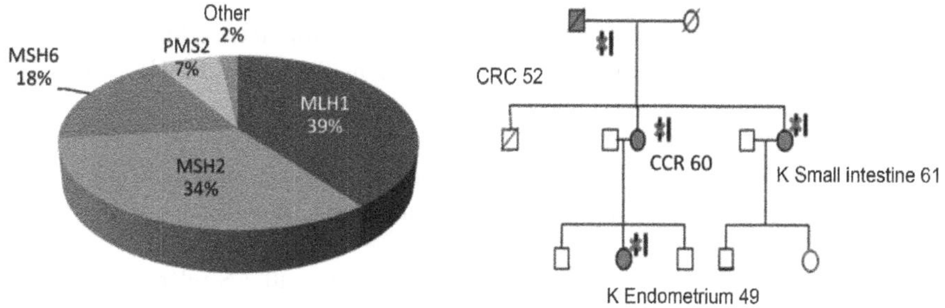

a) b)

Figure 2.1. *Autosomal dominant transmission Lynch syndrome (MMR +/–): (a) involvement of different MMR genes in Lynch syndrome (percentage of mutations predisposing to LS in a given MMR gene); (b) example of a family with Lynch syndrome (association of colorectal and endometrial cancers). K: cancer, CRC: colorectal cancer, the numbers indicate the age of patient at diagnosis. For a color version of this figure, see www.iste.co.uk/boukhatem/oncogenetics.zip*

Constitutional MMR deficiency (MMRd) syndrome results from the biallelic inheritance of mutations affecting the MMR genes: MLH1, MSH2, MSH6 or PMS2 and is characterized by early-onset malignancies. Fewer than 150 cases have been reported in the literature over the past 20 years.

2.3. Genes

The proteins produced by MLH1, MSH2, MSH6 and PMS2 form heterodimeric complexes, which play an essential role in DNA repair. The complex formed between MSH2-MSH6 (MutSα) recognizes and binds to single nucleotide base pair mismatches and small insertion–deletion anomalies, after which a second heterodimer complex between MLH1-PMS2 (MutLα) binds to MutSα and recruits exonuclease-1, triggering the *long segment excision* of newly synthesized DNA in the vicinity of the mismatched DNA. DNA repair enzymes rapidly release DNA allowing resynthesis of the excised segment, usually correctly.

The loss of MMR DNA activity leads to the rapid accumulation of mutations (hypermutated genome) and possibly mutations in genes that are the effectors of carcinogenesis.

2.4. Genotype–phenotype correlations

Genotype–phenotype correlations are established because cancer risk depends on the mutated MMR gene. Patients with mutations in the MLH1 and MSH2 genes have significant abnormalities in DNA repair and therefore have a higher oncogenic risk than patients with other MMR mutations, such as PMS2 and MSH6, who have a low risk of extracolonic cancer.

Some studies report that MSH2-mutated patients develop more multiple primary and extracolonic cancers and have less CRC than MLH1 patients.

PMS2 mutations carriers show the lowest risk for all LS-related cancers. In addition, carriers of EPCAM mutations exhibit mosaic-specific cell inactivation of MSH2, and therefore have a different tumor profile compared to carriers of mutations in MMR genes; in particular, the risk of endometrial cancer in EPCAM deletion carriers is significantly lower than in MMR gene mutation carriers.

In the majority of cases of MTS, germline mutations in the MSH2 and MLH1 genes have been identified in patients. Ninety percent of patients with MTS are reported to have mutations in the MSH2 gene, with less than 10% having abnormalities in MLH1.

Germline mutations in the other MMR genes are rarely associated with MTS (MTS cases with MSH6, PMS2 or MLH3 mutations have been reported).

In the case of Lynch syndrome associated ovarian cancer (LSAOC), a lifetime ovarian cancer (OC) risk of 20% for MLH1 mutations, 24% for MSH2 mutations and 1% for MSH6 mutations has been reported.

CMMR-D patients with MLH1/MSH2 mutations have an earlier age of onset of malignancy (mean age 3.5 years) than patients with biallelic mutations MSH6 and PMS2, respectively (mean age 9 years). The prevalence of hematologic tumors is higher in patients with MLH1 or MSH2 mutations, while patients with biallelic mutations MSH6 and PMS2 have a higher incidence of brain tumors and other tumors associated with LS.

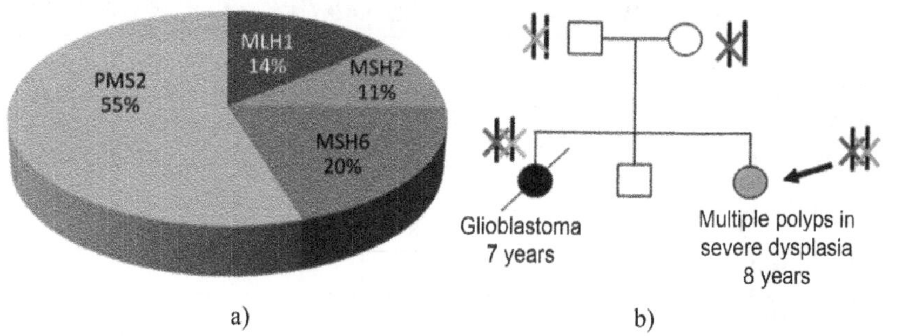

Figure 2.2. *CMMRD syndrome (constitutional MMR deficiency) recessive autosomic transmission (MMR –/–): (a) participation of different MMR genes in CMMRD; (b) example of a family with a CMMRD (both parents are each carriers of a mutation in the same MMR gene). For a color version of this figure, see www.iste.co.uk/boukhatem/oncogenetics.zip*

With regard to the risk of gastric cancer (GC), a study reported some predilection for carriers of the MSH2 mutation to develop such a cancer (standardized SIR incidence ratio: 6.1 for MSH2 vs. 2.9 for MLH1).

2.5. Penetrance and survival

The genotype deficient in MMR genes (MMR deficient) is associated with a lifetime cancer risk of 58–75% with frequent observations of the development of synchronous/metachronous tumors. Colorectal cancer and EC predominate with estimated cumulative risks of 10–74% and 15–71%, respectively.

Upper tract urothelial cancer (UTUC) is considered the third most common cancer in LS with a cumulative lifetime risk of 2.9–28%, depending on the individual case.

Cancers of the ovaries, stomach, hepatobiliary tract, small intestine, brain and skin have been shown to develop with increased incidence in LS, while for breast cancer, prostate cancer, PC and sarcoma, risk estimates are inconclusive.

Some studies have estimated the cumulative risk of LSAOC to be 2% at age 40, 15% at age 60 and 20% at age 80. Compared to sporadic OC, an earlier age of onset of LSAOC has been reported. The estimated median age of LSAOC is 48 years compared to a mean age of 63 years in the general population.

Type of cancer	All (%)	MLH1 (%)	MSH2 (%)	MSH6 (%)	PMS2 (%)	EPCAM (%)
Colorectal	10–75	25–70	30–60	10–22	10–20	70
Endometrial	14–71	14–54	20–52	34–71	15	12
Ovarian	1–20	4–15	5–17	1–15	/	/
Gastric	1–13	4–11	2–14	1–10	/	/
Small intestine	1–12	4–10	1–8	0–3	/	/
Pancreatic	1–6	/	/	/	/	/
Prostate	4–10	/	/	/	/	/
Urinary tract	2–15	1–10	2–15	1–15	/	/

Table 2.2. *Estimated lifetime cancer risks in Lynch syndrome by gene*

2.6. Long-term prevalence of cancer in LS patients

Based on the monitoring of a total of 3,119 LS patients (1,723 women and 1,396 men), and a total of 24,475 cumulative years of monitoring, the cumulative lifetime incidence of various types of cancer in patients aged 25–75 years was calculated. The cumulative incidence (risk) at the age of 75 years for CRC was: 46%, 43% and 15%; for EC: 43%, 57% and 46%; for OC: 10%, 17% and 13%; for cancers of the upper gastrointestinal tract (gastric, duodenal, bile duct or pancreatic): 21%, 10% and 7%; for cancers of the urinary tract: 8%, 25% and 11%; for prostate cancer: 17%, 32% and 18%; and for brain tumors: 1%, 5% and 1%, for carriers of mutations in the MLH1, MSH2, and MSH6 pathways, respectively.

OC occurred mainly before menopause. In retrospect, cancers of the upper gastrointestinal tract, urinary tract and prostrate occurred mainly at older ages.

An adapted summary of the cumulative impact is presented in Table 2.3.

	Cumulative impact in % (+95% CI)			
Organ	MLH1	MSH2	MSH6	PMS2
Any cancer	75.8 (68.5–83.2)	80.4 (69.8–90.9)	60.9 (42.7–79.0)	52.1 (0.1–100.0)
Colorectal cancer	45.8 (37.8–53.9)	43.0 (33.2–52.8)	15.0 (3.3–26.6)	0
Gynecological cancers	49.8 (40.5–59.0)	65.7 (52.2–79.1)	54.0 (34.6–73.4)	26.4 (0.8–51.9)
Cancer of the upper gastrointestinal tract	21.4 (15.6–27.1)	10.2 (4.1–16.3)	6.6 (0–14.8)	0
Urinary tract cancer	8.0 (4.3–11.7)	24.9 (16.6–33.2)	11.0 (1.7–20.3)	0
Breast	12.0 (6.7–17.3)	11.5 (4.6–18.4)	13.3 (2.2–24.4)	55.9 (0.0–100.0)
Prostate	16.9 (8.5–25.3)	31.6 (11.7–51.5)	18.3 (0.0–44.4)	37.9 (0.0–95.9)
Brain	1.0 (0.0–2.4)	5.3 (0.2–10.3)	1.4 (0.0–4.2)	0

Table 2.3. *Cumulative incidence of cancer in 75 year old patients with Lynch syndrome*

In the same cohort of LS patients in the above-mentioned study, the percentage of survivals was estimated.

Five-year survival was 96% for colon cancer and 75% for rectosigmoid cancer. The corresponding 10-year survival was 88% and 70%, respectively. The 5-year survival for EC was 93% and 83% for OC, and the corresponding 10-year survival was 93% and 74%, respectively.

Overall 5-year survival for prostate cancer was 100%, bladder 93%, urethra 85%, duodenum 67%, stomach 61%, bile duct 29%, brain 22% and pancreas 0%. Carriers of mutations in the PMS2 pathway had a lower risk of cancer.

With respect to GC risk, a study from the Dutch Hereditary Cancer Registry estimated a standardized incidence ratio (SIR) of 3.4 (95% CI: 2.1–5.2) for carriers of LS mutations compared to the general population, with an absolute risk of 8% for males and 5.3% for females. A study from the Australian Colon Cancer Registry estimated the 10-year risk of gastric and hepatobiliary cancer at 1% (95% CI: 0.2–2), with an SIR of 5.65 (95% CI: 2.32–9.69).

A more recent retrospective cohort study combining data from the German and Dutch national registries cited cumulative GC risks close to 6.7% and 2.6%, with SIRs as high as 9.8 and 7.2 for men and women, respectively. There appears to be no aggregation of GC cases among LS families.

The cumulative risk of developing a brain tumor at 70 years of age would be 1.2% for MSH2 mutation carriers and lower (<1) for MLH mutation carriers. Although the lifetime risk of brain tumors in LS families is low compared to many other tumors, the risk of brain tumors is unequivocally high compared to the general population; the calculated increase is between four and six times.

In published series of LS-associated brain tumors (mainly in MLH1 or MSH2 mutation carriers), the mean age at diagnosis ranged from 33 to 53 years.

NOTE.– Prostate, urinary tract, gastric, duodenal, biliary tract and pancreatic cancers occur frequently in elderly LS patients.

Prostate and urinary tract cancers occur mainly in carriers of mutations in the MSH2 pathway.

Cancers of the upper gastrointestinal tract occur primarily in carriers of mutations in the MLH1 pathway.

OC occurs primarily in younger women, which is in contrast to OCs in carriers of mutations in the BRCA1/2 pathway and in the general population.

Survival is very poor for bile duct and PCs, intermediate for stomach, duodenum and urinary tract cancers and good for prostate cancer.

With the exception of endometrial and prostate cancers, typical LS cancers have not been diagnosed in carriers of mutations in the PMS2 pathway.

2.7. Mode of transmission

These predispositions are usually inherited in an autosomal dominant mode and are often characterized by early onset of disease. It should be noted that some variants of LS (TS and CMMR-D) have autosomal recessive transmission.

2.8. When to suspect LS

LS should be suspected in patients whose tumors show signs of MSI and meet diagnostic criteria through clinical guidelines such as the Amsterdam criteria.

The Amsterdam I criteria emphasize aspects of the patient's personal and family history that are more restrictive and consider only CRC, while the Amsterdam II criteria are broader criteria that also consider other cancers associated with LS.

2.8.1. *Amsterdam II criteria*

The Amsterdam II criteria resulting from the revision of the Amsterdam I criteria can be stated as follows:

– at least three relatives with LS-related cancer (colorectal, endometrial, small bowel, ureteral or excretory kidney cancer);

– one should be a first-degree relative of the other two;

– at least one should be diagnosed before the age of 50;

– familial APC should be excluded in case of CRC;

– tumors must be verified by pathological examination.

2.8.2. *Criteria to help identify families with LS*

Other general criteria applicable to any syndrome of genetic predisposition to cancer can also help identify families with LS:

– the age of cancer reporting is earlier than in the general population;

– primary cancers segregate through the family tree;

– survival differs from the norm for the specific cancer;

– tumors are associated with distinctive pathological features;

– germline mutations should be identified in affected family members.

The National Comprehensive Cancer Network (NCCN) recommends that all CRC patients must have their tumors universally tested for MSI phenotype to correctly identify patients with LS.

The detection sensitivity of patients with a deleterious constitutional mutation of an MMR gene in the CRC population is increased if other parameters, not limited to the Amsterdam criteria and predictive of the presence of an MSI+ tumor phenotype, are taken into account (Bethesda criteria). The presence of at least one of these criteria is an indication to test for an unstable MSI+ tumor phenotype.

2.8.3. *Revised Bethesda criteria*

The Bethesda criteria (established in 1997 and revised in 2004) that increase the sensitivity of detection of patients with a deleterious constitutional mutation in an MMR gene are as follows:

– CRC diagnosed before the age of 50;

– two synchronous or metachronous cancers of the broad spectrum of LS, regardless of the age of diagnosis, in the same patient;

– CRC with the anatomopathological characteristics of MSI+ cancers (large lymphocyte infiltrate, Crohn's-like lymphocyte response, signet ring cell carcinoma, large mucinous component) at an age below 60 years;

– CRC with at least one first-degree relative with Lynch spectrum cancer and, at least in one case, with an age at cancer diagnosis of less than 50 years;

– CRC with at least two first- or second-degree relatives with Lynch spectrum cancer, regardless of cancer diagnosis age.

2.8.4. *Spectra and syndromes*

LS presents a wide variety of tumor spectra that can be divided into four groups as follows:

– "narrow" LS tumor spectrum: colon, endometrium, ovaries and excretory urinary tract;

– "wide" LS tumor spectrum: small intestine, stomach, bile ducts, glioblastomes, etc.;

– TS: colon and SNC tumors (glioblastoma, medulloblastoma, ependymoma);

– MTS: sebaceous skin tumors, keratoacanthomas, deep visceral tumors (colon, endometrium, digestive tract, urinary tract, etc.).

Colon cancer patients with a high MSI histology (associated with criteria such as tumor infiltrating lymphocytes, Crohn's-like lymphocyte response, signet ring cells or spinal cord growth pattern) and who are under 60 years of age should also be tested.

DEFINITION.– Keratoacanthoma *is a fast-growing dome-shaped skin tumor that usually occurs on areas of the body exposed to the sun, in particular the head, neck, arms, legs and the backs of the hands. Keratoacanthomas often start in a hair follicle. They may resemble squamous cell skin cancer, but they are usually benign and rarely spread to other parts of the body.*

2.9. Tumors

2.9.1. *Colorectal cancer*

Lynch-associated CRCs can be distinguished from sporadic MSI-H CRCs in that Lynch-associated tumors are almost always devoid of the somatic mutations in the BRAF gene and the hypermethylation of the MLH1 promoter, both characteristic of the so-called "serrated neoplastic pathway".

Lynch-associated CRCs behave differently than sporadic CRCs, which has significant implications for clinical management. With respect to oncology treatment, the histopathological and molecular characteristics of Lynch-associated CRCs are associated with differences in prognosis and therapeutic responses. These differences in prognosis and therapeutic responses are partly explained by the fact that the DNA MMR system is involved in the triggering of chemotherapy-induced cell death, which is absent in non-MSI CRCs.

These tumors resulting from defective DNA MMR are also hypermutated and generate neo-antigenic peptides that can induce a strong host immune response. Patients with MSI have also been shown to be more likely to respond to treatment by blocking the immune checkpoint (anti: PD-1, PD-L1 or CTLA-4).

Histopathological examination of Lynch-associated CRCs often reveals abundant lymphocytes infiltrating the tumor.

CRCs associated with LS are usually on the colon right side and are more often multifocal. In addition, colon polyps in patients with LS develop at a younger age, are smaller, and are more likely to be villous polyps.

The prognosis for CRC patients who have (MMRd) tends to be better, stage by stage, compared to cancers with a functional DNA MMR pathway.

2.9.2. *Endometrial cancer*

In addition to family history and age criteria, histomorphological characteristics have been suggested as screening parameters for LS-related ECs. MMR morphology is defined as undifferentiated histology, tumor infiltrating lymphocytes (440 for 10 high-magnification fields), peritumoral lymphocytes and an origin in the lower uterine segment. However, only 42% of LS-related ECs may have one or more of these characteristics.

Histologically, endometrial tumors with MSI or MMRd are predominantly endometrioid; however, non-endometrioid subtypes have been described. These tumors typically have tumor-infiltrating lymphocytes and peri-tumor lymphocytes. In addition, a pattern of invasion called microcystic, elongated, fragmented and lymphovascular space invasion has also been associated with MMRd endometrial tumors.

There is some evidence to suggest that EC in MSH2 carriers has more histologic features than non-endometrioid tumors, such as clear cell carcinoma, papillary serous uterine carcinoma and malignant mixed Mullerian tumors, although the majority of these tumors are still of the endometrioid histologic type.

In addition, endometrial carcinomas with mixed endometrioid and clear cell histology are frequently deficient in MMR proteins. This finding has implications for the identification of patients with potential LS.

2.9.3. *Bladder and urothelial tract*

A study examined four histological features to determine if they were useful in identifying tumors for which the MSI test was performed (pushing borders, tumor-infiltrating lymphocytes, reverse growth pattern and high nuclear grade without pleomorphism). A summary of the results of this study is presented in Table 2.4.

Features	Lynch (%)	Sporadic (%)	Sensitivity (%)	Specificity (%)	*P*-value
Pushing borders	86 (12/14)	53 (107/201)	86	47	0.03
High nuclear grade without pleomorphism	71 (10/14)	/	71	56	0.06
Moderate to marked intratumoral lymphocytes*	36 (5/14)	9 (18/201)	36	91	0.0045
Reverse growth	21 (3/14)	10 (20/201)	21	90	0.19

*Defined as ≥ 20 lymphocytes/10 high-magnification fields.

Table 2.4. *Histological characteristics of tumors in relation to Lynch syndrome*

As with CRC, a similar relationship may exist between cancers deficient in MMR and immune checkpoint inhibitors (patients with MSI have also been shown to be more likely to respond to treatment with immune checkpoint blockades). This is particularly important because two immune checkpoint inhibitors, atezolizumab and nivolumab, have recently been approved by the US FDA for use in the treatment of metastatic urothelial carcinoma.

2.9.4. *Dermatological tumors*

Sebaceous gland neoplasia with possible keratoacanthomas is observed in MTS.

Sporadic sebaceous tumors occur most often in the head and neck area, while lower neck sebaceous neoplasms are associated with MTS. Lesions are yellow papules or nodules that may have central umbilication and ulceration and include sebaceomas, sebaceous adenomas/epitheliomas/carcinomas, sebaceous differentiated basal cell epitheliomas and seboacanthomas.

Sebomatricomas have been associated with MTS and can be used as an indicator of this syndrome.

DEFINITION.– Sebomatricoma *or* sebaceoma *is a term that encompasses all benign neoplasms with sebaceous differentiation. It is a rare benign cutaneous neoplasm with sebaceous differentiation.*

2.9.5. *Pancreatic tumors*

It has been described that pancreatic tumors developed by LS patients often have a typically medullary appearance, with prominent lymphocyte infiltration and MSI.

Although LS has been clearly associated with pancreatic ductal adenocarcinoma, no clear connection has been established with pancreatic neoplastic precursor lesions in these patients.

Only a few recent publications have shown that intraductal papillary mucinous neoplasms may be related to LS and therefore that these lesions should be carefully considered when screening patients.

2.9.6. *Tumors of the ovary*

LSAOC is rare. However, recent studies have shown that the predominant histological subtype among LSAOC is endometrioid adenocarcinoma (53%), followed by high-grade serous adenocarcinoma (17%), mixed tumors (11%) and clear cell carcinoma (11%). It should be remembered that in non-LS and BRCA-associated OCs, high-grade serous cancers predominate.

2.9.7. *Brain tumors*

Brain tumors associated with LS can be of various histological types, the most common being glioblastoma and astrocytoma (see Table 2.1). Since the MSI phenotype is generally rare in brain tumors, its presence may indicate the presence of a germline mutation in one of the MMR genes. Note that a clear qualitative difference in the MSI profile was evident when glioblastoma from a TS patient and colon cancer from an affected relative were compared. The glioblastoma had smaller allelic shifts that may make the MSI phenotype more difficult to discern and which supports the idea that the type of MSI varies in tumors of different histological derivation.

DEFINITION.– Astrocytoma *is a tumor that starts in the brain or spinal cord in small star-shaped cells called astrocytes.*

2.10. Monitoring

2.10.1. *Colorectal cancer risks*

The monitoring of CRC in MMR mutation carriers could be effective and significantly more cost effective. Due to the early age of CRC onset in LS and the predominance of proximal colon involvement, full colonoscopy should be initiated before the age of 20–25 years. It is because of the accelerated carcinogenesis in LS CRCs compared to non-MMR CRCs (CRC in 2–3 years compared to 8–10 years for non-MMR CRCs) that colonoscopy should be started at this early age (20–25 years).

Chromoendoscopy (coloration with indigo carmine or other dye during endoscopy to improve the detection of polyps) is preferred to conventional colonoscopy because of its advantages (inexpensive equipment and easily performed procedure). However, more sophisticated techniques exist, such as virtual colonoscopy, which have the advantage of not being as invasive (see Figure 2.3).

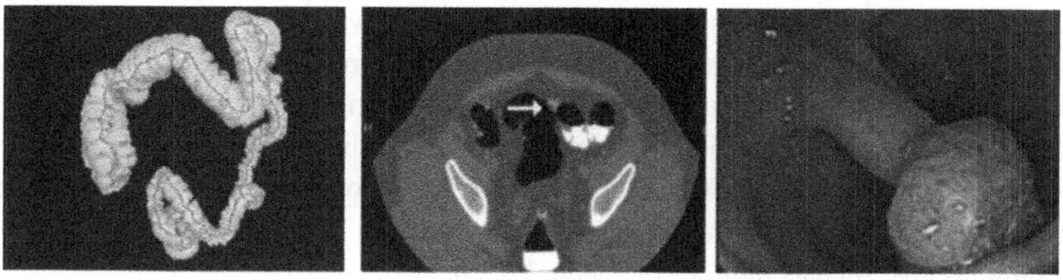

a) b) c)

Figure 2.3. *Virtual colonoscopy can create a three-dimensional (3D) anatomical model of the colon using volumetrically acquired CT scan data*

COMMENT ON FIGURE 2.3.– *(a) Virtual colonoscopy is capable of graphically reproducing a three-dimensional (3D) image of the anatomy of the patient's colon; (b) the arrow points to a pedunculated polyp in the sigmoid colon; (c) optical colonoscopy confirmed the presence of a 1.5 cm pedunculated polyp, located 50 cm from the anus.*

Prophylactic colectomy as part of risk management in LS patients is highly controversial. It was pointed out that there are no prospective clinical studies evaluating the potential benefit of prophylactic colectomy in LS.

Clinical practice guidelines for LS from the US Multi-Society Task Force on CRC include colectomy with ileorectal anastomosis as primary treatment for LS patients with CRC or non-removable colon neoplasia by endoscopy.

In all cases, a balance between cancer prevention and considerations of discomfort and complications following these procedures should be maintained.

DEFINITION.– *A* colonoscopy *is an examination used to detect changes or abnormalities in the large intestine (colon) and rectum. During a colonoscopy, a long flexible tube (colonoscope) is inserted into the rectum. A tiny video camera at the end of the tube allows the doctor to see the inside of the entire colon.*

DEFINITION.– Colectomy *is a surgical procedure to remove all or part of the colon. When only part of the colon is removed, it is called a partial colectomy.*

2.10.2. *GC risks*

A family history of GC may increase the likelihood of an abnormal gastroscopy. In recent years, chromoendoscopy has emerged as a new endoscopic tool for the detection of preneoplastic gastric lesions in LS (*Helicobacter pylori* infection, atrophic gastritis and intestinal gastric metaplasia). Most expert bodies currently advise against routine screening, but suggest that it should be considered in certain higher risk individuals. It has been advocated that gastric screening in asymptomatic individuals should be restricted to high-risk groups, based on family history and possibly ethnicity. The NCCN guidelines do not recommend routine gastroscopy monitoring in patients with LS, but recommend that it should be considered for certain groups, such as families of Asian descent.

DEFINITION.– *A* gastroscopy *is a procedure in which a thin, flexible tube called an endoscope with a video camera is used to examine the inside of the esophagus, stomach and the first part of the small intestine (duodenum).*

2.10.3. *Risks of endometrial and ovarian cancer*

Due to the limited effectiveness of endometrial and, in particular, ovarian cancer monitoring, prophylactic hysterectomy and bilateral adnexectomy may be considered (in the absence of maternity plans and/or approaching 40 years of age) in LS patients. Such surgery has been shown to result in a significant reduction in endometrial and ovarian cancer in LS patients.

The incidence of very early age peaks for OC (30–49 years) and brain tumors (50–69 years) and increased incidence rate ratios for urothelial cancer after age 50 and in MSH2 mutation carriers should be considered in future monitoring strategies for patients with LS.

Surveillance can be tailored to individual women because MSH6 carriers have a high risk of EC but a lower risk of OC. Women with PMS2 mutations appear to have the lowest risk of OC.

DEFINITION.– *The term* hysterectomy, *in the literal sense of the term, simply refers to the removal of the uterus and sometimes the cervix. When the uterus and cervix are removed, it is called a total hysterectomy. When only the uterus is removed, it is called a partial hysterectomy.*

DEFINITION.– *The* endometrium *is the internal epithelial layer of the uterus with its mucous membrane. It has a basal layer and a functional layer; the functional layer thickens and is then lost during menstruation.*

2.10.4. *Risks to the bladder and urothelial tract*

Patients with LS-associated urothelial upper tract cancers should be strictly monitored for recurrences of this type of cancer and for all other cancers included in the LS spectrum. For cancers of the urinary tract, a urinary check-up and imaging cytology (ultrasound or urogram with computerized tomography) should be offered annually from the age of 30–35 years.

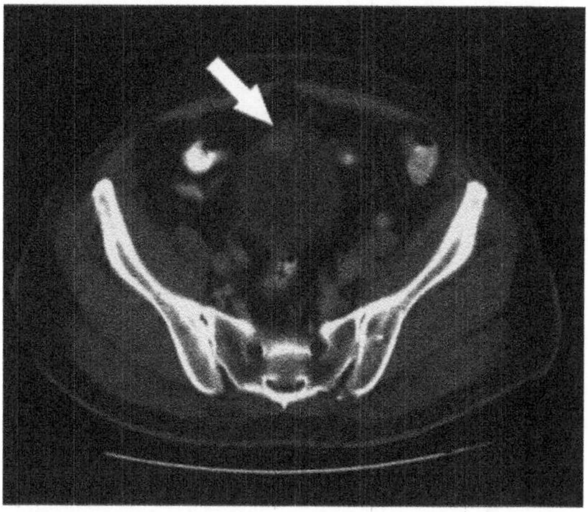

Figure 2.4. *Bladder cancer. Computed tomography (CT) scan of the bladder showing bladder cancer (arrow)*

2.10.5. *Risks of dermatological tumors*

For sebaceous tumors, there are no clear recommendations, but patients with LS and their relatives should have regular dermatological examinations, especially in cases of MTS.

2.10.6. *Risks for other types of cancer*

For other cancers, no routine monitoring is clearly recommended beyond what is advised for the general population.

NOTE.– The recent report (see section 2.6) that provided for the first time a prospectively observed empirical result of health care for the elderly with LS and with stratification by affected MMR pathway should be considered before revising risk management guidelines to reflect this stratification (after validation by other studies).

3

Neurofibromatosis

3.1. Introduction

The term neurofibromatosis refers to a group of disorders characterized by an autosomal dominant mode of transmission with high rates of spontaneous mutation and multiple neurofibromas or neurilemmomes. Neurofibromatosis 1 (generalized neurofibromatosis) accounts for approximately 95% of all neurofibromatosis cases, although several additional subtypes (e.g. neurofibromatosis 2, schwannomatosis, and so on) have been described.

3.2. Neurofibromatosis type 1

3.2.1. *Introduction*

Multiple café au lait spots as well as axillary and inguinal freckles in addition to choroidal freckles are the most visible signs of neurofibromatosis type 1 (NF1). Other manifestations of the disease include multiple cutaneous neurofibromas, Lisch nodules of the iris and about half of people with NF1 have plexiform neurofibromas, but most are internal and are only detectable by imaging techniques. At least 50% of people with NF1 have learning disabilities. Less frequent but potentially more severe manifestations are also described. They include optic nerve glioma and other gliomas of the central nervous system (CNS), malignant tumors of the peripheral nerve sheath, scoliosis, tibial dysplasia and vasculopathy.

3.2.2. *Prevalence*

The prevalence of this disease is about one in 2,500–7,800 people. About half of the cases are familial (hereditary) in origin.

Constitutional Oncogenetics,
Noureddine BOUKHATEM.

3.2.3. *When to suspect NF1*

NF1 should be suspected in individuals with any of the following criteria:

– six or more café au lait spots with a maximum diameter > 5 mm in prepubescent individuals and > 15 mm in postpubescent individuals;

– two or more neurofibromas (any type) or a single plexiform neurofibroma;

– freckles in the axillary or inguinal regions;

– optical glioma;

– two or more Lisch nodules (hamartomes of the iris);

– a distinctive bone lesion such as sphenoidal dysplasia or tibial pseudarthrosis;

– a first-degree relative with NF1.

DEFINITION.– Hamartoma *is a benign (non-cancerous) growth consisting of an abnormal mixture of cells and tissues normally present in the area of the body where the growth occurs.*

3.2.4. *Tumors*

Neurofibromas are benign Schwann cell tumors that can affect virtually any nerve in the body. Cutaneous neurofibromas develop in virtually all people with NF1 and increase in number with age (although the increase in size is very slow). Plexiform neurofibromas develop in about half of the cases with NF1.

Peripheral nerve sheath malignancies are the most common malignant neoplasms associated with NF1, occurring in approximately 10% of affected individuals. Compared to the general population, peripheral nerve sheath malignancies tend to occur in individuals with NF1 at a younger age, often in adolescence or early adulthood.

It appears that NF1 individuals most at risk of developing peripheral nerve sheath malignancies are those who have a deletion of the entire NF1 gene, have benign subcutaneous neurofibromas or have a high burden of benign internal plexiform neurofibromas compared to NF1 individuals who do not have these characteristics.

The most common neoplasms besides benign neurofibromas in patients with NF1 are optic nerve gliomas and brain tumors.

Optic gliomas in people with NF1 are generally asymptomatic and remain so throughout life. The majority of these lesions seem to regress spontaneously (their prevalence decreases from about 20% in young children to less than 5% in older adults with NF1).

The clinical course in patients with optic gliomas tends to be less severe in patients with NF1 than in those without NF1. A second CNS glioma occurs in 17–20% of individuals with NF1 who have optic gliomas.

Brain stem and cerebellar gliomas in individuals with NF1 may also follow a less aggressive course than in those without NF1.

Leukemia (especially juvenile chronic myeloid leukemia) and myelodysplastic syndromes are rare in children with NF1, but still much more common than in children without NF1. A variety of other tumors may also be seen more frequently than expected in individuals with NF1, including rhabdomyosarcomas, pheochromocytomas, gastrointestinal stromal tumors, glomal tumors and retinal vasoproliferative tumors. Women with NF1 have a significantly increased risk of developing and dying from breast cancer before the age of 50. People with NF1 may also have an increased risk of other types of cancer.

DEFINITION.– Pheochromocytoma *is a tumor that forms in the center of the adrenal gland resulting in overproduction of adrenaline. Pheochromocytomas are usually benign (not cancerous), but can cause high blood pressure, severe headaches, heart palpitations, flushing, nausea and vomiting.*

DEFINITION.– Rhabdomyosarcoma *is a rare cancer that forms in soft tissue, especially skeletal muscle tissue or sometimes in hollow organs such as the bladder or uterus. Rhabdomyosarcoma can occur at any age, but most often affects children.*

3.2.5. *Gene*

Mutations in the NF1 gene induce NF1. The NF1 gene encodes a protein called neurofibromin. This protein is produced in many different cells, including nerve cells and specialized cells surrounding nerves (oligodendrocytes and Schwann cells). Neurofibromin acts as a tumor suppressor and functions as a negative regulator of the RAS signal transduction pathway.

NF1 is a RAS GTPase activating protein and thus facilitates the inactivation of RAS. In cells lacking NF1, RAS activation is not inhibited by NF1, which induces transcriptional changes and proliferative signaling via the RAF-MAP kinase pathway and prosurvival signaling via the PI3K-mTOR axis. Therefore, loss or mutation of NF1 gene is an important step in tumorigenesis in NF1 patients.

It is not known how mutations in the NF1 gene lead to other features of NF1, such as café au lait spots and learning disabilities.

3.2.6. *Genotype–phenotype correlations*

NF1 is characterized by extreme clinical variability. This variability is not only observed between unrelated individuals or among affected individuals within the same family, but even within a single person at different times of life.

Only a few clear correlations have been observed between particular pathogenic alleles of NF1 and clinically consistent phenotypes.

The deletion of the entire NF1 gene is associated with a large number of cutaneous neurofibromas and their early appearance, more frequent and severe cognitive abnormalities, somatic proliferation, large hands and feet, and facial dysmorphia.

A 3 bp phase deletion of exon 17 (c.2970-2972 delAAT) (nomenclature of the NF Consortium, exon 22 of the NCBI nomenclature) is associated with pigmentary characteristics typical of NF1, but not with cutaneous or surface plexiform neurofibromas.

Multiple café au lait spots, learning disabilities, short stature and pulmonary stenosis, but with the absence of clinically apparent cutaneous neurofibromas or plexiform neurofibromas, are associated with all of the many missense variants affecting the NF1 Arg1809 codon in exon 29 (NF Consortium nomenclature, exon 38 of the NCBI nomenclature).

The extreme clinical variability of NF1 suggests that random events are important in determining the phenotype of affected individuals.

3.2.7. *Penetrance*

NF1 penetrance evolves rapidly from null penetrance at birth to full penetrance after childhood and in early adolescence.

3.2.8. *Mode of transmission*

As with most genetic predispositions to cancer, the mode of transmission of NF1 is the autosomal dominant mode.

3.2.8.1. *Risk to family members*

3.2.8.1.1. Parents of a proband

Approximately 50% of people diagnosed with NF1 have an affected parent. Approximately 50% of people diagnosed with NF1 have this condition as a result of a *de novo* NF1 pathogenic variant.

3.2.8.1.2. Related to a proband

The risk to siblings of the proband depends on the clinical status of the proband's parents. If one parent is affected, the risk to siblings is 50%; a sibling who inherits a pathogenic variant NF1 will develop characteristics of NF1, but the disease may be considerably more (or less) severe in affected siblings than in the proband (variable penetrance).

If none of the parents of an individual with NF1 meet the criteria for a clinical diagnosis of NF1 after a thorough medical history, physical examination and ophthalmological examination, the risk to relatives of this affected individual having NF1 is low, but higher than in the general population due to the possibility of germline mosaicism (germline mosaicism for NF1 pathogenic variants has been demonstrated).

3.2.8.2. *Lineage of a proband*

Each child of an individual with NF1 has a 50% chance of inheriting the pathogenic variant NF1.

Penetrance is 100%; thus, a child who inherits a pathogenic variant NF1 will develop characteristics of NF1, but the disease may be considered more (or less) severe in an affected child than in the affected parent (variable penetrance).

Other family members may be affected. The risk to other family members depends on the status of the applicant's parents: if a patient's parent is affected, other family members may be at risk.

3.2.8.3. *Problematic cases related to genetic counseling*

There is a possibility of multiple *de novo* pathogenic variants in the same family (three different NF1 pathogenic variants have been reported in one family and two different NF1 pathogenic variants have been reported in another family).

The hypothesis of a *de novo* pathogenic variant in families must be considered. When no pathogenic variant has been identified in the parents of an autosomal dominant disease progenitor and in the absence of clinical evidence of the disorder in the parents, the pathogenic variant is likely *de novo*. However, non-medical explanations, including alternative paternity or maternity (e.g. with Medically Assisted Procreation) or undisclosed adoption, may also be considered.

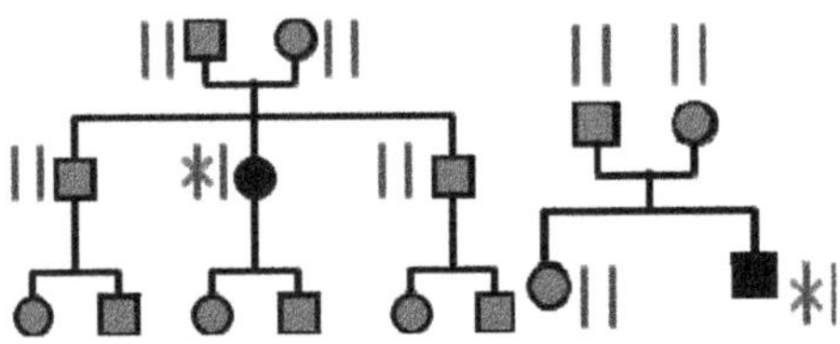

Figure 3.1. De novo *mutations are more or less frequent according to the genes in the dominant predispositions (30% of cases of familial adenomatous polyposis syndromes and 3% of cases of Lynch syndrome are due to* de novo *mutation or neomutations). Individuals (black circle and square) have parents who do not have the mutation they have*

3.2.9. *Monitoring*

The American Academy of Pediatrics and various other groups have developed guidelines for monitoring NF1 patients. The recommendations are as follows:

– annual physical examination by a physician familiar with the individual and the disease;

– annual ophthalmologic examination in early childhood; less frequent examination in older children and adults;

– regular developmental assessment by screening questionnaire (in childhood);

– regular blood pressure monitoring;

– other examinations (e.g. magnetic resonance technology (MRI)) only as indicated on the basis of clinically apparent signs or symptoms;

– monitoring of those with CNS, skeletal system or cardiovascular system abnormalities by an appropriate specialist.

Because of the increased risk of developing breast cancer before the age of 50 in NF1 women, the National Comprehensive Cancer Network (NCCN) guidelines recommend that mammography be performed annually and that breast MRI be considered between the ages of 30 and 50 in women with NF1. However, the effectiveness and cost effectiveness of this screening has not yet been demonstrated.

Rare cases of concomitant BRCA and NF1 mutations have been reported. Awareness of the possible concomitance of NF1 and BRCA1 mutations is important in identifying the genetic origin of early-onset breast cancer in patients with NF1 in order to allow early detection of cancers and to reduce breast cancer morbidity and mortality in these patients.

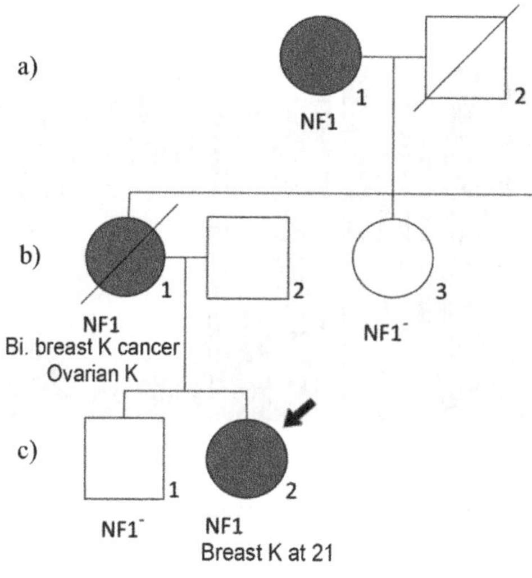

Figure 3.2. *Family tree showing index case c2 (black arrow) diagnosed with invasive breast cancer at age 21 and with NF1 at birth. DNA testing reveals the presence of mutations in the NF1 and BRCA1 genes. The mother of index case b1 has NF1 and has developed bilateral breast cancer and ovarian cancer*[1]

3.3. Neurofibromatosis type 2

3.3.1. *Introduction*

Neurofibromatosis type 2 (NF2) is an autosomal dominant genetic disease caused by mutations in the NF2 gene (OMIM 607379). It is characterized by the

1 See Jeon *et al*. (2015).

development of multiple tumors of the nervous system and meninges, as well as eye and skin lesions, resulting in high morbidity and reduced life expectancy. A characteristic feature of this disorder is the presence of one to three bilateral vestibular schwannomas (BVS) in more than 90% of NF2 adults.

DEFINITION.– *A* schwannoma *is a type of nerve sheath tumor. It is the most common type of benign peripheral nerve tumor in adults. It can occur anywhere in the body at any age.*

Other types of schwannomas are also described in NF2 patients: schwannomas of other cranial, spinal and cutaneous nerves. Tumor development is also reported: cranial and spinal meningiomas and/or other tumors of the CNS, including ependymomas and low-grade astrocytomas.

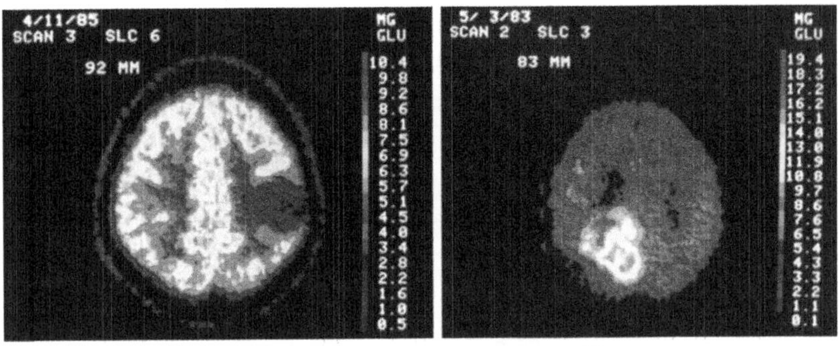

a) b)

Figure 3.3. *Astrocytomas. For a color version of this figure, see www.iste.co.uk/boukhatem/oncogenetics.zip*

COMMENT ON FIGURE 3.3.– *(a) PET (positron emission tomography) scan: astrocytoma (grade 1). A PET scan of a 17-year-old girl with a brain tumor classified as grade 1 astrocytoma. The PET scan indicates that the tumor does not metabolize excess glucose and is therefore benign; (b) a PET scan of a 62-year-old man with a brain tumor classified as grade III astrocytoma. The PET scan shows an increase in the metabolic rate of glucose, illustrated by the irregular bright white area in the center of the scan. PET scans allow doctors to tell if a tumor is malignant without the need for a surgical biopsy.*

DEFINITION.– Ependymoma *is a type of brain tumor that begins in the cells lining the central canal or ventricles of the spinal cord. Ependymoma can also form in the choroid plexus (the tissue in the ventricles that produces cerebrospinal fluid). It is also called an* ependymal tumor.

3.3.2. *Prevalence*

The prevalence is about one in 60,000. The incidence at birth has been estimated at one in 33,000.

3.3.3. *When to suspect NF2*

The diagnosis is confirmed in the following cases:

– bilateral masses of the vestibule (eighth cranial nerve) observed with appropriate imaging techniques (e.g. CT or MRI) plus a family history of NF2;

– unilateral vestibular schwannoma plus two of the following: neurofibroma, meningioma, glioma, schwannoma and juvenile posterior subcapsular lenticular opacity.

The diagnosis is likely in case of:

– multiple meningiomas (two or more) and unilateral vestibular schwannoma;

– two of the following conditions: neurofibroma, glioma, schwannoma and cataract.

3.3.4. *Tumors*

3.3.4.1. *Vestibular schwannomas*

Vestibular schwannomas are the most common tumors in NF2 and are usually present bilaterally, although they are often of different sizes; one usually predominates over the other.

Similarly, intracranial meningiomas, spinal cord tumors or skin tumors may occur prior to the development of vestibular schwannomas and account for approximately 20–30% of presentations. Hearing loss due to vestibular schwannomas is the tell-tale symptom in 60% of adults and 30% of children.

3.3.4.2. *Intracranial meningiomas*

This is the second most common type of tumor in NF2 patients and can occur anywhere in the cranial cavity, but is most often localized in the convexities. It can also occur around the base of the skull and in the optic nerve region.

DEFINITION.– Meningioma *is a type of slow-growing tumor that forms in the meninges (thin layers of tissue that cover and protect the brain and spinal cord). Meningiomas usually occur in adults.*

3.3.4.3. *Spinal tumors*

Up to 90% of NF2 patients have spinal tumors. Extramedullary meningiomas and schwannomas are the most common types of tumors. Ependymomas of the spinal cord are also frequently observed.

3.3.5. *Gene*

NF2 is caused by mutations in the NF2 gene, coding for neurofibromin-2 or schwannomin (SCH), also known as the ezrin-radixin-moesin like (ERM) protein, located on chromosome 22q12.2.

The NF2 gene has 17 exons encoding Merlin protein, a 69 kDa protein with 595 amino acids. Merlin consists of three domains, a trilobal FERM (4.1-ezrin-radixin-moesin) domain on the amino-terminal side, an alpha-helical domain and a carboxy-terminal domain. There are two isoforms, an active and closed non-phosphorylated form and an open and inactive phosphorylated form.

Phosphorylation occurs at serine 518 and is catalyzed by cyclic protein kinase A-AMP and p21-activated kinases. This prevents the protein from refolding leading to its inactivation and relocalization.

Dephosphorylation is catalyzed by the myosin phosphatase-1d of the protein phosphatase-1. Merlin is localized at the cell membrane/cytoskeleton interface and appears to have a number of different roles involving the interaction between cell membrane proteins and cytoskeletal or intracellular proteins (F-actin, b2-spectrin, Rho guanosine triphosphatase), the organization of cell membrane proteins (epidermal growth factor receptor EGFR and CD44) and cell adhesion (E-cadherin, b1-integrin).

The details of these roles are not clear at present, but all result in downstream regulation of cell proliferation via a number of pathways including the MAPK pathway and the phosphoinositide-3 kinase (PI3K) pathway.

3.3.6. *Genotype–phenotype correlations*

Germinal mutations occur throughout the first 15 exons, but not in exons 16 and 17 of NF2. The predominant mutations are nonsense mutations on the CpG islets, but all other forms of mutations can occur, including multiexon deletions and deletions of the whole gene. There is a relatively strong phenotypic correlation between the phenotype and the position of the NF2 germline mutation.

Individuals with truncating mutations (nonsense/frameshift) induce earlier symptoms, more meningiomas and spinal tumors and carriers of such mutations die younger. Truncated mutations in exon 1 and 14/15 show less severe symptoms. The splice site mutations are less deleterious than truncated mutations and there is also a positional effect with more severity correlating with more proximal mutation positions. Large deletions/duplications are intermediate, with missense mutations being associated with the less severe form.

3.3.7. *Penetrance*

NF2 usually occurs in early adulthood, although less severe phenotypes may appear much later. Penetrance is variable and can reach almost 100% by the age of 60.

3.3.8. *Mode of transmission*

As with most genetic predispositions to cancer, the mode of transmission of NF2 is the autosomal dominant mode.

3.3.9. *Risks to family members*

Approximately 50-60% of patients have no family history and represent *de novo* mutations. In *de novo* patients with BVS, 70% will have the mutation in all their cells because the mutation will have occurred prezygotically.

However, in the remaining 30% there is somatic mosaicism (the mutation occurs postzygotically and not all cells carry the mutation).

In *de novo* patients with unilateral vestibular schwannoma, the incidence of mosaicism is 60%. These patients often have less severe symptoms and have a less than 50% risk of transmitting the disease to their offspring.

The risk of transmission depends on the degree of mosaicism. A *de novo* NF2 mosaic patient with BVS has a one-eighth risk of transmitting the disease to their children. The risk drops to one-twelfth if the patient has unilateral vestibular schwannoma. For children who have received the mutation from a parent (in whom the mutation appeared *de novo* or not), the transmission is 50% from the second generation onwards (constitutional mutation). Children of mosaic cases generally have more severe symptoms than the affected parent.

3.3.10. *Monitoring*

The first step in a monitoring program is to conduct presymptomatic testing of at-risk patients.

Since early detection of tumors is effective in improving the clinical management of NF2 patients, screening for NF2 in the children of affected patients can begin at birth with the search for cataracts. If no cataracts are found, presymptomatic genetic testing, if possible, should be considered.

In children of affected parents, screening can begin at birth with the search for cataracts. Formal screening should begin at 10 years of age with a cranial and spinal MRI and an audiological assessment. Below the age of 20, these examinations should be performed every 2 years. Beyond 20 years of age, when tumor growth becomes slower, a check-up every 3–5 years is acceptable. These examinations may be discontinued at the age of 40. If a person has a proven mutation but has not yet shown symptoms of NF2, cranial imaging should be performed annually with spinal imaging every 3 years.

For those at 1–19% risk, including those with unilateral vestibular schwannoma between the ages of 20 and 30, the investigation should include cranial and spinal MRI, audiology, and ophthalmologic and dermatologic assessments at baseline and between 18 and 20 years of age. Additional cranial MRI scans should be performed 5, 10 and 20 years after the initial assessment. If there is no evidence of NF2 at this stage, the risk of the disease development is less than 1%.

Once diagnosed, an annual MRI of the head is performed. MRI of the spine is usually performed every 3 years in patients with spinal tumors unless there are new symptoms. In patients who have not developed a spinal tumor, MRI should be done every 5 years.

3.4. Schwannomatosis

3.4.1. *Introduction*

Schwannomatosis is characterized by the predisposition to developing multiple non-vestibular schwannomas and, more rarely, meningiomas. Multiple schwannomas are non-intradermal, cranial, spinal and peripheral. Other features of NF2 such as cataract and ependymoma are absent.

In contrast to patients with NF1 who show characteristic dermatological signs and patients with NF2 who present cranial eighth nerve dysfunction at a young age, patients with schwannomatosis have non-specific symptoms that may delay consultation or imaging and thus diagnosis.

3.4.2. *Prevalence*

Schwannomatosis is a rare disease with an estimated prevalence of about 1:40,000 to 1:70,000. This is probably an underestimated prevalence, as it is difficult to identify those affected.

3.4.3. *When to suspect schwannomatosis*

Patients with schwannomatosis most often develop symptoms in the second or third decade of life, but a formal diagnosis is usually delayed by about 10 years. Patients usually suffer from pain (46%), a mass (27%) or both (11%). Pain is the most frequently reported symptom by patients, with 68% of patients suffering from chronic pain. Schwannomas usually affect the spine (74%) and peripheral nerves (89%), however schwannomas of the cranial nerve (mainly trigeminal) are rare (8%).

Segmental schwannomatosis, presumably due to genetic mosaicism, has been reported in approximately 30% of patients. However, detailed studies of suspected segmented patients raise the possibility that segmental schwannomatosis may not be the consequence of genetic mosaicism, but rather a variant of tumor formation.

3.4.4. *Tumors*

Schwannomas affect various regions of the body including the extremities, spinal cord, chest wall and subcutaneous areas.

Vestibular schwannomas are rare in schwannomatosis syndrome. Until recently, the presence of vestibular schwannoma excluded a schwannomatosis diagnosis, but patients with SMARCB1 and LZTR1 germline mutations have been identified (phenotypic overlap between schwannomatosis and NF2).

Meningiomas occur in about 5% of patients with schwannomatosis and have a predilection for the falx cerebri. Families with multigenerational meningiomas and SMARCB1 germline mutations have been reported.

3.4.5. *Genes*

Two major clinical/molecular forms have been characterized so far:

1) schwannomatosis-1 (SWNTS1) [MIM #162091] caused by constitutional (germline) inactivating mutations in the SMARCB1 gene (SWI/SNF related, matrix associated, actin-dependent regulator of chromatin, subfamily B, member 1; MIM #601607) located at 6 Mb centromeric to the NF2 gene at 22q11.23;

2) schwannomatosis-2 (SWNTS2) [MIM #615670] caused by constitutional/ inactivator mutations in the germline of the LZTR1 gene (leucine zipper-like transcriptional regulator 1 gene; MIM #600574).

SMARCB1 codes for an ATP-dependent SWI/SNF nuclear chromatin remodeling protein, which is part of a complex that:

1) reduces the repressive structures of chromatin, allowing the transcriptional machinery to access its targets more efficiently;

2) binds to HIV-1 integrase and enhances its DNA joining activity (SWI/SNF is a tumor suppressor also involved in the genesis of malignant rhabdoid tumors).

SMARCB1 acts as a tumor suppressor by regulating the cell cycle and inducing senescence. In addition, SMARCB1 and the SWI/SNFs regulate lineage age-specific gene expression as well as embryonic stem cell programming.

LZTR1 encodes a protein that is a member of the BTB-kelch superfamily that is located exclusively in the Golgi network where it can help stabilize the Golgi complex.

LZTR1 mutations have been identified in several cancers, and the LZTR1 gene functions as a tumor suppressor in glioblastoma, where biallelic mutations have been reported.

3.4.6. *Genotype–phenotype correlations*

Germline mutations in the SMARCB1 gene have been identified in 40–50% of families with familial schwannomatosis and in 10% of individuals with sporadic schwannomatosis.

The SWNTS1 phenotype (as a result of mutations in the SMARCB1 gene) is characterized by several schwannomas and extra-axial/extramedullary meningiomas (as well as a unilateral vestibular schwannoma).

The SWNTS2 phenotype (as a result of mutations in the LZTR1 gene) is characterized by a late onset of the disease (20–60 years of age) and schwannomas affecting various regions of the body including the extremities, spinal cord, chest wall and subcutaneous regions.

In addition, vestibular schwannomas occur at a low frequency in individuals with LZTR1 mutations.

Inherited mutations found in familial schwannomatosis are more likely to be non-truncated mutations (missense or splice site), which predominate at each end of the gene and are potentially hypomorphic.

In 2013, mutations in the LZTR1 gene were identified in a high proportion of cases of SMARCB1-negative schwannomatosis with NF2 gene loss in their tumors. This finding was confirmed in independent cohorts of patients.

Mutations in a second rhabdoid tumor locus, SMARCA4 (Brg1), also a component of the SWI/SNF complex, have been reported in a small number of patients.

3.4.7. *Penetrance*

Data on the penetrance of schwannomatosis are limited. Penetrance is generally incomplete and is less than 100% for both SMARCB1- and LZTR1-related schwannomatosis. Reduced penetrance has been reported more frequently in individuals with LZTR1-related schwannomatosis.

3.4.8. *Mode of transmission*

Familial schwannomatosis accounts for 15% of reported cases and is autosomal dominant.

Initial assessment of patients who have or are at risk of schwannomatosis should include tests to confirm a diagnosis (usually by excluding NF1 and NF2).

The medical history should include questions about auditory and vestibular function, focal neurological symptoms, skin tumors or hyperpigmented lesions, epilepsy, headaches and visual symptoms.

Given the incomplete penetrance of schwannomatosis, the absence of symptoms in first-degree relatives cannot be considered as an indication that these individuals do not carry the responsible germline mutation.

3.4.9. *Monitoring*

The management of patients with schwannomatosis is mainly symptom oriented. Pain is the characteristic feature of this disorder and remains the most difficult to treat. Surgery should be reserved for patients with symptomatic tumors or rapidly expanding lesions. Surgery is the treatment of choice for symptomatic schwannomas and, in many patients, can relieve local pain or symptoms resulting from compression of surrounding tissue.

4

Familial Adenomatous Polyposis

4.1. Introduction

Familial adenomatous polyposis (FAP) accounts for approximately 1% of all colorectal cancers (CRCs). FAP syndromes can be divided into classical FAP and attenuated FAP (AFAP), MUTYH-associated polyposis (MAP), NTHL1-associated polyposis (NAP) and polymerase proofreading-associated polyposis (PPAP).

4.1.1. *FAP*

The disease is caused by mutations in the APC (adenomatous polyposis coli) gene that lead to the development of hundreds to thousands of adenomas (polyposis) in the colon and rectum at an abnormally young age. Without treatment (if the colon is not removed), one or more of these adenomas would invariably become malignant with almost 100% penetrance. The mode of transmission is autosomal dominant.

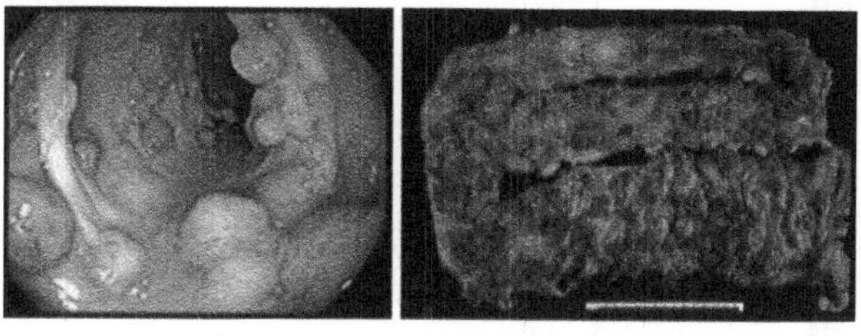

a) b)

Figure 4.1. *(a) Countless polyps are present throughout the colon and rectum, ranging in size from 3 to 8 mm, as shown here during colonoscopy; (b) many polyps are present on a surgically removed colon*

4.1.2. *AFAP*

AFAP is a milder form of classical FAP with fewer polyps (< 100) and a later age of onset of polyps/cancers. The disease is due to mutations in the APC gene. The mode of transmission is autosomal dominant.

4.1.3. *MAP*

MAP is an autosomal recessive inherited disease caused by germline mutations in the MUTYH gene (which encodes an enzyme called MYH glycosylase, involved in DNA repair).

4.1.4. *NAP*

NAP is a second hereditary recessive form of polyposis discovered recently (2015). It is caused by mutations in the base excision repair (BER) gene, NTHL1. To date, only 12 affected individuals have been described. Most had between 10 and 50 adenomas and two-thirds had already developed CRC.

4.1.5. *PPAP*

This is an autosomal dominant inherited disease caused by germline mutations in the POLE and POLD1 genes.

NOTE.– We will deal with hamartomatous polyposis elsewhere (Peutz–Jegher syndrome and juvenile polyposis syndrome).

Name	Abbreviation	Genetics	Transmission	Clinical manifestations
Classic familial adenomatous polyposis	FAP	APC gene germline mutations	Autosomal dominant	100–1,000 colorectal polyps occurring early to mid-30s (usually 16 years) and rapidly increasing; almost 100% risk of CRC if untreated
Attenuated familial adenomatous polyposis	AFAP	APC gene germline mutations	Autosomal dominant	< 100 colorectal polyps (usually 30) between 40 and 70 years of age (mean 55 years); estimated 70% risk of CRC by age 80 years

Name	Abbreviation	Genetics	Transmission	Clinical manifestations
MUTYH-associated polyposis	MAP	MUTYH biallelic germline mutations	Autosomal recessive	Usually < 100 polyps at an average age of 50 and high risk of CRC; associated with malignant tumors of the duodenum, ovary, bladder and skin
Polyposis associated with NTHL1	NAP	Homozygous or heterozygous germline mutations of NTHL1	Autosomal recessive	The number of polyps is unknown, because it is of a recently discovered association, but a wide spectrum of cancers has been observed (CRC, endometrium, duodenum, skin, breast, pancreas and others); multiple primary tumors in all patients
Polymerase proofreading-associated polyposis	PPAP	Germline mutations of POLE or POLD1	Autosomal dominant	Number of polyps unknown, also recently discovered; associated multitumoral phenotypes such as colon/pancreas/ovary/small intestine and colon/ovary/endometrium/brain

Table 4.1. *Summary of different types of polyposis adenomatous syndromes*

4.2. Prevalence

4.2.1. *FAP*

The prevalence of FAP is around 1 in 10,000 live births. FAP also accounts for about 1% of all CRCs with an equal distribution among men and women.

4.2.2. *MAP*

So far, more than 100 different variants of MUTYH have been described. Two European founder mutations, c.536A > G (p.Tyr179Cys) in exon 7 and c.1187G > A (p.Gly396Asp) in exon 13, predominate in the Western world and are found in 70–90% of MAP patients depending on the geographical region.

Several other founding mutations were reported (see Table 4.2). The heterozygous frequency in normal controls, in a British cohort and in Australian, Canadian, and American cohorts was 1–2%.

The reported heterozygous frequency for 35 pathogenic (likely) MUTYH mutations, including the two founder mutations, is slightly less than 0.8%.

Population studies show that MAP is responsible for 0.4% of all colon cancers and 1–2% of familial and early (i.e. < 50 years of age) CRCs.

Country	Variation at DNA level	Variation at protein level
Western Europe	c.536A > G c.1187G > A	p.Gly396Asp p.Tyr179Cys
Pakistan	c.312C > A	p.Tyr104*
Northern Europe	c.1147delC	p.Ala385Profs*23
Germany	c.1214C > T	p.Pro405Leu
Italy	c.1437_1439del	p.Glu480del
India, United Kingdom	c.1438G > T	p.Glu480*
Spain, Portugal, Tunisia	c.1227_1228dup	p.Glu410Glyfs*43
Spain, France, Brazil	Deletion of exon 4–16	/
Japan, South Korea	c.1118C > T c.857G > A	p.Ala373Val p.Gly286Glu

Table 4.2. *MUTYH founder mutations in patients of different ethnic backgrounds; *the amino acid should switch to a stop codon (Ter)*

4.2.3. *NAP*

The prevalence of NAP in the European population can be estimated at one in 114,770. The prevalence of pathogenic variants, with the exception of p.Gln90* (nonsense mutation), is extremely low in the European population.

4.2.4. *PPAP*

Approximately 1% of patients with evidence of an inherited form of polyposis carry a suspected pathogenic variant in the exonuclease domains (EDM) of both genes (POLE and POLD1). POLE EDM is also somatically mutated in ~1% of CRC and ~8% of endometrial cancers.

4.3. When to suspect FAP

The development of many polyps (> 10) and their occurrence at very young or relatively young ages along with the familial aggregation of CRCs are the main indicators of polyposis syndromes. Determining the type of predisposition syndrome is dependent on the identification of the gene responsible for the constitutional mutation causing the syndrome.

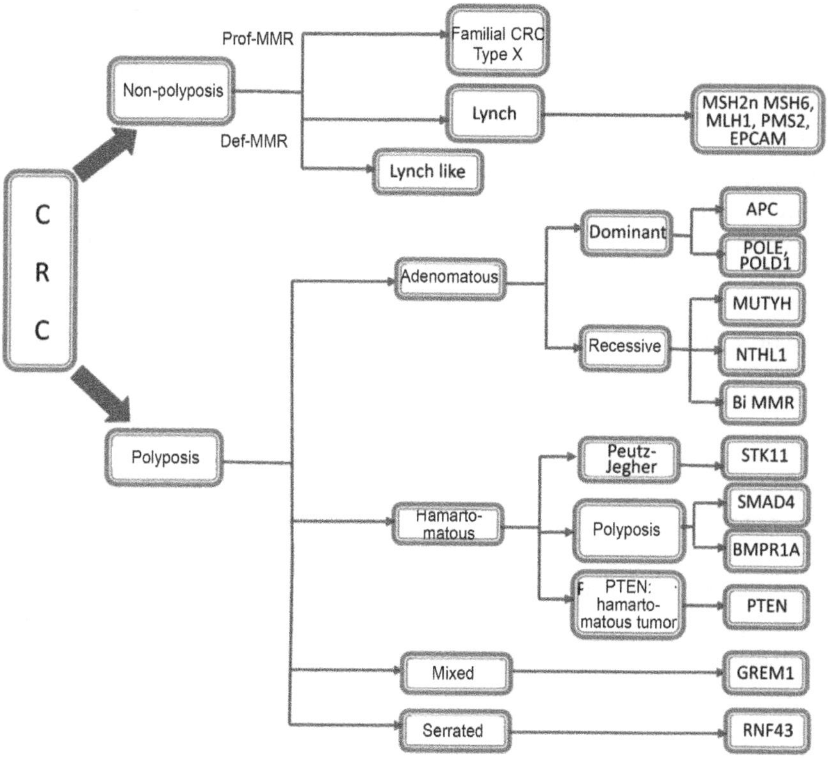

Figure 4.2. *Classification of colorectal cancer predisposition syndromes*

4.4. Tumors

4.4.1. *FAP*

Patients with FAP almost inevitably develop CRC at an average age of 40–50 years (if the colon has not been surgically removed). In 70–80% of cases, CRC is located on the left side of the colon.

The duodenum and the periampullary region is the second most common region where adenomas will develop and prevalence varies between 33% and 92%.

Other gastrointestinal manifestations include fundic gland polyps (which occur in approximately 90% of FAP patients and are usually benign).

Extracolonic manifestations are frequent, but rarely malignant and include desmoid tumors (benign soft tissue tumors that can be fatal due to progressive invasion into the surrounding tissues); skin lesions such as fibroids, lipomas and sebaceous and squamous cell cysts (Gardner syndrome, phenotypic variant of FAP); congenital hypertrophy of the retinal pigmentary epithelium (CHRPE); and lesion causing discoloration of the fundus.

Low-grade adeno-carcinoma has been described in these lesions: brain tumors (mainly medulloblastoma, described in Turcot syndrome); hepatoblastoma; dental abnormalities; pancreatic, thyroid, gallbladder and bile duct; and adrenal gland cancers.

DEFINITION.– Hepatoblastoma *is a type of liver tumor that occurs in infants and children.*

DEFINITION.– Lipoma *is a benign (not cancerous) tumor made up of fat cells.*

4.4.2. *MAP*

The diagnosis of colorectal polyposis in patients with MAP is made at an average age of 48 years. Colorectal carcinoma is present in approximately 60% of MAP patients at the time of diagnosis. As in Lynch syndrome, adenomas appear to progress rapidly to carcinomas.

In addition to CRC, higher risks for several other malignant and benign tumors have been described. It was shown that the prevalence of duodenal polyposis in the MAP cohort was 17% and the cumulative risk of duodenal carcinoma was 4%. A significantly increased risk of bladder cancer (HR = 19; SIR[1] = 7) and ovarian cancer (HR = 19; SIR = 6) was reported. Skin cancer (SIR = 2.8), including melanomas, basal cell carcinomas and squamous cell carcinomas, and a significant increase in breast cancer incidence (SIR = 3.0; 95% CI = 1.5–5.3) were also reported. Other tumors found in MAP patients included sebaceous gland tumors present in approximately 2% of patients.

---

1 Standardized incidence ratio.

The characteristics of MAP carcinomas are somewhat comparable to those of Lynch and sporadic MMR-deficient tumors, with often proximal localization in the colon, secondary colon cancers, a high number of lymphocytes infiltrating the tumors and an often relatively mucinous histotype.

4.4.3. *NAP*

All patients described so far have developed adenomas, ranging from one tubulo-tubular adenoma to more than 50 adenomas. Adenomatous polyps appear to be present in all affected individuals, but striated and mixed polyps also appear. In addition to CRC, several other malignancies have been identified, both in the gastrointestinal tract and in extracolonic tissues: meningiomas, bladder cancer and basal cell carcinoma, endometrial cancer and breast cancer are among them.

4.4.4. *PPAP*

Overall, the PPAP phenotype appears to be characterized by attenuated adenomatous polyposis of the colorectum (> 80% of POLE and > 60% of POLD1 mutation carriers diagnosed with ≥ 2 adenomas, mean of 16 adenomas), CRC (60–64% of carriers) and probably brain tumors (6%).

Duodenal adenomas were detected in 14 patients with a POLE mutation who underwent upper digestive tract endoscopy. In addition to an intestinal phenotype, the POLD1 phenotypic spectrum includes endometrial and breast tumors.

Unlike Lynch syndrome, cancers appearing in PPAP are generally microsatellite stable.

In view of the observation that POLE-mutated tumors have a surprisingly high density of tumor-infiltrating lymphocytes, which is often accompanied by a Crohn's-like reaction, it has been hypothesized that immunotherapy may lead to the control of tumor growth and has therefore been the main cause of the favorable prognosis of these tumors.

4.5. Genes

4.5.1. *APC*

APC is a tumor suppressor gene that plays a central role in the Wnt signaling pathway. APC, located at locus 5q21-22, consists of 15 coding exons (the number of exons has been increased to 18 after identification of two APC promoter regions) and the size of the coding region is 8,532 bp, corresponding to a protein comprising 2,843 amino acids.

APC plays a central role in the Wnt signaling pathway, particularly with respect to the degradation of β-catenin in the cell cytoplasm. If APC is mutated, the β-catenin-Tcf complex is not repressed and leads to the constitutive activation of several genes and oncogenes controlling cell growth and division.

4.5.2. *MUTYH*

The MUTYH gene is a BER gene located on chromosome 1p34.1. There are three major MUTYH transcripts (α, β and γ) and at least 10 isoforms of the MUTYH protein (429–549 amino acids). The longest transcript, NM_001128425.1 (alpha 5), is used as the coding sequence reference.

MUTYH is the only protein that recognizes an 8-oxo-7,8-dihydro-2'-deoxyguanosine (8-oxodG) incorporated in front of an adenine (8-oxoG: A, mismatch) and excises the undamaged (but misincorporated) adenine base using a flip-flop mechanism, thus preventing transversion (G:C > T:A) from occurring at the next replication cycle.

4.5.3. *NTHL1*

The NTHL1 gene is located on chromosome 16p13.3. The NTHL1 protein, similar to MUTYH, is involved in repair by basic excision. The NTHL1 protein is a BER protein involved in the repair of a number of oxidized bases, although it is not clear at this time which oxidation product is covered by NTHL1.

4.5.4. *POLE and POLD1*

POLE and POLD1, respectively, encode the main subunits of polymerase ε and polymerase δ. The polymerases δ and ε, together with all other eukaryotic polymerases, belong to the family of B DNA-dependent polymerases. Their main function is to replicate the genome. The false incorporation of nucleotides by the polymerases of the B family members is low (10^{-4} to 10^{-5}) and the fidelity of replication is enhanced by the proofreading function of these enzymes, which further reduces replication errors by about 100 times.

4.6. Genotype–phenotype correlations

4.6.1. *FAP*

In families with FAP, considerable variability in disease expression is observed within and between relatives with identical APC mutations and it has been shown that the higher the number of colorectal adenomas, the higher the risk of CRC.

Patients with mutations in the mutation cluster region (MCR) of the APC gene, located between codons 1286 and 1513, generally have a poorer prognosis (with earlier disease reporting) than patients with mutations outside this region.

Germline mutations in codon 1309 are associated with more severe symptoms, while less severe forms with less than 100 adenomas and later ages of onset (AFAP) are associated with regions before codon 157, between codons 312 and 412 and after codon 1595 of the APC gene.

In AFAP, APC mutations are mainly observed in three sections of the gene (first exons, exon 9 and at the distal end of the APC).

CHRPE has been associated with mutations between codons 457 and 1444 and susceptibility to desmoid tumors is correlated with mutations between codons 1395 and 2000 of the APC gene.

A wide phenotypic variation was observed in patients with identical germline mutations, strongly suggesting the existence of FAP modifier alleles.

4.6.2. *MAP*

Functional studies have shown that the p.Y179C mutation (of the MUTYH gene) has a worse effect on glycosylase function than the p.G382D mutation. Indeed, individuals with homozygous p.Y179C have a more severe phenotype than homozygous p.G396D, showing a younger age of onset (mean age of CRC diagnosis of 46 years compared to 58 years). A recent study in Italian patients showed an even more severe phenotype for MAP patients with the p.Glu480del mutation than those with p.Gly396Asp and/or p.Tyr179Cys, because they had a younger age at diagnosis of polyps. To date, these genotype–phenotype correlations do not support differences in monitoring.

4.6.3. *PPAP*

Although the prospect of a genotype–phenotype correlation of POLE is suggested, the small amount of data precludes any significant conclusion.

4.7. Penetrance

4.7.1. *FAP*

If left untreated (if the colon is not removed), one or more of the adenomas invariably become malignant with almost 100% penetrance.

4.7.2. *MAP*

Estimates indicate that the risk of CRC in patients with MAP is approximately 43% at age 60 and the lifetime risk is presumed to be close to 100% in the absence of timely colon monitoring. The high number of adenomas is likely responsible for this increased risk of cancer.

4.7.3. *PPAP*

The scarcity of phenotypic data results in a lack of clarity regarding the penetrance of cancers related to the POLE and POLD1 mutations.

4.8. Mode of transmission

For FAP and PPAP, transmission is autosomal dominant, while for MAP and NAP it is autosomal recessive.

4.9. Monitoring

4.9.1. *FAP*

Current recommendations strongly encourage initiation of colonic surveillance at 10–12 years of age for individuals with a genomic APC mutation compatible with profuse and intermediate polyposis (also known as classical FAP) and in late adolescence for AFAP.

Unlike colon monitoring, current guidelines for upper digestive tract monitoring do not distinguish between the different genotypes of APC; basic upper endoscopy with lateral vision is recommended from 20 to 25 years of age with a frequency ranging from 3 to 48 months, depending on the extent of duodenal polyposis.

The diagnosis of cancer via colonoscopy is a clear indication for colectomy in patients with FAP or PPAP. Colectomy is also considered appropriate in patients with FAP who are monitored for large adenomas (>1 cm), advanced histology of polyps, or an increased polyps load that is no longer manageable by colonoscopy (usually >20).

The main surgical options available are total colectomy with ileo-rectal anasatomosis or proctocolectomy with ileo-anal anastomosis. Even in cases of colectomy, the risk of developing cancers in the remaining parts of the colon and rectum is not zero and monitoring of these areas is recommended.

DEFINITION.– Anastomosis *is a procedure for connecting healthy sections of tubular structures in the body after the diseased part has been surgically removed.*

DEFINITION.– Proctocolectomy *is the surgical removal of the rectum and all or part of the colon. It is a widely accepted surgical method for ulcerative colitis and FAP.*

4.9.2. *Monitoring of extracolonic cancer*

There is a risk of duodenal cancer of up to 12% in patients with FAP and approximately 65% of patients have duodenal adenomas. The prevalence and high risk of cancer development warrants regular monitoring, and it is recommended that screening begin before the age of 25–30 years based on the Spigelman classification system.

The guidelines suggest that duodenectomy preserving the pancreas may be considered in patients with Spigelman stage IV.

Extracolonic monitoring is suggested for the stomach and thyroid. Malignancies of the pancreas, biliary tract and gallbladder have been reported in FAP. However, due to the lower risk of developing these tumors, there are currently no associated standard screening guidelines.

4.9.3. *MAP*

The frequency of monoallelic mutations of MUTYH in the general population is approximately 1–2%. These individuals will not develop polyposis, but large population studies have shown a slightly increased risk (OR = 1.1–1.2 in meta-analyses) for the development of CRC.

Carriers of MUTYH heterozygous mutations in a MAP family should therefore be screened based on their family history. This includes participation in population-based CRC screening or colonoscopy every 5 years starting at age 45 when CRC is present in first-degree relatives without MAP.

4.9.4. *NAP*

Currently, the same monitoring program as for MAP has been recommended. Annual breast and endometrial screening from age 40 onwards may be added for women in the future (subject to confirmation by observation of additional carriers to establish more accurate risks for specific extracolonic tumors).

4.9.5. *PPAP*

There is a lack of consensus on how PPAP patients should be treated clinically, again reflecting the scarcity of phenotypic data and the lack of clarity regarding cancer penetrance. However, the manifestation of the colorectal adenomas described in the second decade and the increased risk and multiplicity of CRCs in the third decade of these patients' lives make colonoscopic monitoring of these patients advisable. It has been proposed that colonoscopy be performed every 1–2 years starting at age 18.

Whether or not prophylactic surgery is necessary will depend on the patient's phenotype, which will also determine the choice of the required prophylactic surgery. This decision regarding surgery can be based on the phenotypic parameters that have been used in FAP. Using this guide, it is likely that for most patients with PPAP, prophylactic surgery will be required: a colectomy and ileorectal anastomosis would be appropriate.

The high prevalence of duodenal adenomas and cases of duodenal cancer suggest that surveillance of the upper gastrointestinal tract is also recommended, as in patients with FAP. This would involve initiation of upper GI endoscopy (usually with a side-view endoscope) from the age of 25 years, with the monitoring interval being the shortest as determined by the Spigelman stage and the presence or absence of ampullary pathology.

The need for extra-intestinal monitoring has been suggested as well as adding screening for endometrial cancer from the age of 40 for women with POLD1.

For families where a pathogenic mutation is identified, predictive genetic testing may be performed. But there is no consensus as to the age at which this should be offered. Given the phenotypic data, it would seem reasonable to propose predictive testing around the age of 14–16 years.

5

Endocrine Neoplasia

5.1. Introduction

Children and adolescents with neuroendocrine tumors have a very high probability of having an underlying hereditary predisposition to multiple endocrine neoplasia (MEN) syndromes, including MEN syndrome type 1 (MEN1), MEN2A and MEN2B, MEN4, and hyperparathyroid jaw tumor (HPT-JT) syndromes.

Each of these autosomal dominant syndromes is the result of a specific germinal mutation in single genes: MEN1 is due to pathogenic variants of the MEN1 gene (11q13), MEN2A and MEN2B are due to pathogenic variants of the RET gene (10q11.21), MEN4 is due to pathogenic variants of the CDKN1B gene (12p13.1), and HPT-JT syndrome is due to pathogenic variants of the CDC73 gene (1q25).

5.1.1. *MEN1*

MEN syndrome type 1 (MEN1, MIM * 131100) is a disorder in which different combinations of endocrine and non-endocrine tumors may present extremely varied phenotypic clinical profiles. Considerable phenotypic variability in tumor type and age at diagnosis has been reported, even within the same family, where affected members share the same genetic mutation.

5.1.2. *MEN2*

Predisposition to MEN type 2 (MEN2 * OMIM 171400) is caused by activating mutations in the germline of the proto-oncogene RET. The MEN2 syndrome occurs in three clinically distinct subtypes with medullary thyroid carcinoma (MTC) as the most common manifestation. The three subtypes of MEN2 differ in terms of incidence, genetics, age of onset, association with other diseases, aggressiveness of MTC, and prognosis.

5.1.2.1. *MEN2A*

MEN2A syndrome is the most common form and is characterized by MTC associated with pheochromocytoma and/or multiple parathyroid gland tumors in a single patient or the presence of multiple tumor types in several members of a given family.

5.1.2.2. *MEN2B*

MEN2B syndrome is the least common but most aggressive form of MEN2 (5–10% of all cases). It consists of MTC, pheochromocytoma without hyperparathyroidism, and visible physical features such as bumpy lips and tongue (neuromas) and a marfanoid habitus.

5.1.2.3. *FMTC*

Familial MTC (FMTC) is the least morbid form of MEN2. This syndrome accounts for 35–40% of all cases of MEN2. Patients with FMTC have a high predisposition to developing MTC with a very low incidence of other clinical manifestations of MEN2A.

5.1.3. *MEN4*

MEN type 4 (MEN4; OMIM #610755) was first described as a single clinical entity in 2006. However, to date, the lack of sufficient affected patients has limited the ability to generate a complete picture of the syndrome. MEN4 patients appear to have a more restricted phenotype, closer to that of MEN1, with a high incidence of primary hyperparathyroidism (PHPT) (in 100% of patients) and pituitary neuroendocrine tumor (PitNET).

5.1.4. *HPT-JT*

In HPT-JT syndrome (OMIM # 145001), rare individuals or families with PHPT develop ossifying fibroids of the jaw (distinct from the "brown tumors" of hyperparathyroidism) and occasionally parathyroid carcinomas.

5.2. Prevalence

The estimated global prevalence of MEN1 is expected to be between 1:20,000 and 1:500,000, but geographical aggregations due to founding effects have also been reported.

The prevalence of MEN2 in the general population is estimated at 1/40,000.

5.3. When to suspect endocrine neoplasia

The clinical diagnosis of MEN1 is based on the identification of at least two of the major constituent tumors (e.g. parathyroid tumor, islet cell tumor and PitNET). MEN1 is clinically defined when at least two first-degree relatives have a combination of one of the three major endocrine tumors.

MTC is the first neoplastic manifestation in most members of the MEN2 families because of its higher penetrance and earlier onset.

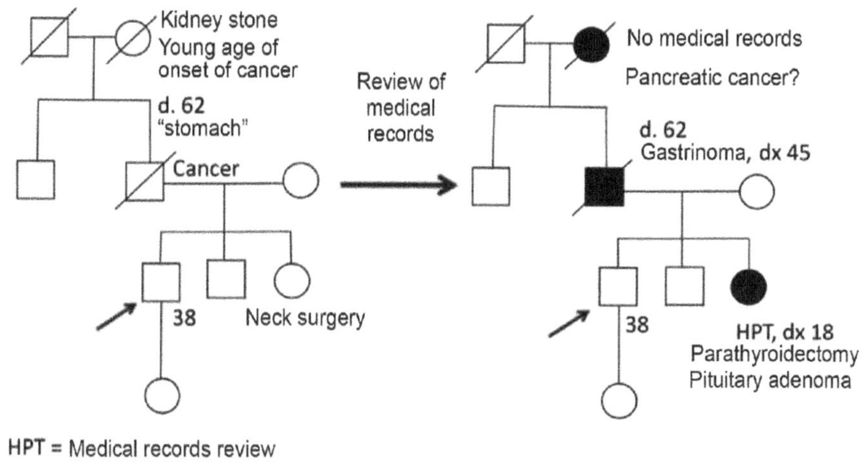

Figure 5.1. *MEN1 pedigree; d.: death; dx: age at diagnosis*

COMMENT ON FIGURE 5.1.– *MEN1 syndrome can be very difficult to identify in a pedigree. The pedigree on the left has been constructed on the basis of self-assessment, and the pedigree on the right represents the same family after a review of available medical records. This pedigree shows some of the characteristics of a family with a deleterious MEN1 mutation over four generations, including family members with hyperparathyroidism, pituitary adenoma, gastrinoma and a suspected pancreatic tumor. Tumors in MEN1 generally occur at an earlier age than their sporadic counterparts.*

DEFINITION.– Gastrinoma *is a tumor that causes an overproduction of gastric acid. It usually begins in the duodenum or pancreatic islets. Rarely, it may also start in other organs, including the stomach, liver, jejunum (the middle part of the small intestine), bile ducts, mesentery or heart. It is a type of neuroendocrine tumor that can metastasize (spread) to the liver and lymph nodes.*

5.4. Tumors

5.4.1. *MEN1*

The original description of the classic P-triad (parathyroid, pituitary, pancreatic) corresponds to (neuro)endocrine, parathyroid, pituitary and pancreatic tumors. Other endocrine tumors associated with MEN1 (corticosteroid and carcinoid tumors) and non-endocrine neoplasms, mainly benign (angiofibromas of the face, collagenomas and others), may also occur.

The tumor spectrum is characterized by:

– PHPT and hypercalcemia resulting from parathyroid (usually multiglandular) adenomas;

– hormone-secreting or non-secreting pancreatic islet tumors (usually gastrinomas and rarely insulinomas, VIPomas, glucagonomas or other neoplasms);

– anterior PitNET, mainly prolactinomas, less frequently growth hormone (GH) secreting adenomas and rarely other PitNETs.

DEFINITION.– Insulinoma *is an abnormal mass that develops in the insulin-producing beta cells of the pancreas. Insulinomas are usually benign (not cancerous).*

DEFINITION.– Prolactinoma *is a non-cancerous tumor (adenoma) of the pituitary gland that overproduces the hormone prolactin. The main effect is a decrease in the levels of certain sex hormones (estrogen in women and testosterone in men).*

DEFINITION.– *A* vipoma *is a tumor of the non-beta pancreatic islet cells secreting vasoactive intestinal peptide (VIP), resulting in a syndrome of watery diarrhea, hypokalemia and achlorhydria (WDHA syndrome).*

Angiofibromas, lipomas and collagenomas are common dermatologic manifestations of MEN1 and adrenal cortical adenomas are identified in 35% of patients with MEN1.

Other minor manifestations of MEN1 include leiomyomas and neoplasms of the central nervous system (including ependymomas and meningiomas).

DEFINITION.– Angiofibroma *is a benign (non-cancerous) tumor composed of blood vessels and fibrous (connective) tissue. Angiofibromas usually appear as small red bumps on the face, especially on the nose and cheeks. Angiofibromas are a type of vascular tumor.*

DEFINITION.– Leiomyoma *is a benign tumor of smooth muscle, usually in the uterus or gastrointestinal tract. It is also called* fibroma.

5.4.2. *MEN2*

MEN2 is characterized by the occurrence of MTC associated with pheochromocytoma and parathyroid adenoma.

MEN2A is characterized by MTC in association with pheochromocytoma and parathyroid tumors, although some families only manifest MTC (i.e. FMTC).

DEFINITION.– Adenoma *is a tumor that is not cancer. It begins in the glandular cells of epithelial tissue (the thin layer of tissue that covers organs, glands and other structures in the body).*

MEN2B patients develop MTC and pheochromocytoma in association with marfanoid habitus, mucosal neurromas, medullated corneal nerve fibers and dysfunction of the intestinal autonomic ganglia. PHPT does not occur in MEN2B.

Pheochromocytoma (PHEO) is associated with both MEN2A and MEN2B. Familial PHEO may also reflect pathogenic germline mutations at other loci, including VHL (Von Hippel-Lindau syndrome), NF1 (neurofibromatosis type 1/von Recklinghausen disease), SDHx (A-D) and TMEM127 or MAX (hereditary PHEO/paraganglioma syndrome).

5.4.3. *MEN4*

The tumor spectrum appears to be narrower and closer to that of MEN1, with a high incidence of mainly PHPT and PitNET (somatotropic, corticotropic and non-functional adenomas).

5.4.4. *HPT-JT*

Tumors are usually parathyroid adenomas, maxillary or mandibular bone fibroids or infrequently parathyroid cancers. Other manifestations include a high rate of benign and malignant uterine tumors and renal abnormalities including cysts, hamartomas and rarely Wilms' tumor.

5.5. Genes

5.5.1. *MEN1*

The MEN1 gene consists of 10 exons encoding a 610 amino acid protein called *menin*. Menin is constitutively expressed and is found mainly in the nucleus of non-dividing cells.

Menin is extremely versatile. It shows no homology with other known proteins and the mechanism by which its loss of function leads to MEN1 is still unclear. Menin is located mainly in the nucleus; it has two conventional nuclear localization signals (NLS) and at least one other non-conventional NLS in its C-terminal. At the nucleus level, menin can associate with chromatin, double-stranded DNA, lysine-specific histone methyltransferases KMT2A and KMT2B2, and components of a transcriptional repressor complex which include histone deacetylases (HDACs).

Menin interacts with transcription factors such as activating protein-1 (AP-1), JunD, nuclear factor-κB (NF-κB), β-catenin, the mothers against decapentaplegic protein belonging to the SMAD family and the estrogen receptor α (ERα). It is also able to bind to cytoskeletal proteins such as vimentin, and to cytoplasmic cell signaling mediators including Akt1/protein kinase B (PKB) and forkhead box protein O1 (FoxO1). Also, menin has been shown to play a role in cell proliferation, apoptosis and maintenance of genome integrity. In addition, the menin/KMT2A complex also regulates the expression of several Hox genes as well as CDKN1B, a gene of which the inactivating mutations cause MEN4.

5.5.2. *RET*

The RET gene has 21 exons and encodes a tyrosine kinase receptor that appears to transduce growth and differentiation signals in several developing tissues, including those derived from the neural crest. The protein consists of an extracellular portion with a ligand binding domain, a cadherin-like domain (Ca^{2+}-dependent cell adhesion) and a cysteine-rich domain close to the cell membrane. It has a single transmembrane domain and an intracellular part with two tyrosine kinase subdomains, TK1 and TK2.

The RET protein is activated during its ligand-induced dimerization. RET is expressed in neuroendocrine cells such as C cells and MTC precursors and in pheochromocytomas. Hereditary MTC is caused by autosomal dominant mutations, such as gain of function, in the protooncogene RET.

5.5.3. *CDKN1B*

CDKN1B encodes the inhibitor of cell cycle progression p27kip1. In tumor tissues, pathogenic variants of CDKN1B appear to be associated with normal levels of transcription, but with low or undetectable protein levels, suggesting reduced translation or protein half-life in pathogenesis. Other variants appear to be associated with functional defects that interrupt binding to interacting partners or disrupt nuclear localization.

5.5.4. *CDC73*

The CDC73 gene (also known as HRPT-2) codes for the parafibromin protein. The syndrome (HPT-JT) results from truncated (80%) or misdirected variants of this gene (CDC73).

5.6. Genotype–phenotype correlations

5.6.1. *MEN1*

There is no apparent genotype–phenotype correlation in MEN1, and no mutational hotspots.

5.6.2. *MEN2*

It has been successfully shown that associations between specific RET mutations and the age of onset and aggressiveness of MTC as well as the presence or absence of other endocrine neoplasms, such as pheochromocytoma or hyperparathyroidism, exist. Thus, 85% of patients with MEN2A have the 634 codon mutation (exon 11, cysteine-rich domain), with mutations of codons 609, 611, 618 and 620 accounting for a further 10–15%. Pheochromocytomas are also detected in about 50% of patients with mutations of codons 634 and 918 and are rarely seen in mutations of exon 10 (codons 609, 611, 618, 620) or exon 15 (codons 791, 804).

Hyperparathyroidism in MEN2A is most commonly associated with mutations in codon 634, particularly the C634R mutation.

All cases of MEN2A associated with Hirschsprung's disease have mutations in exon 10 (codon 609, 611, 618, 620), while patients with MEN2A with cutaneous lichen amyloidosis are associated with mutations in codon 634.

As many as 95% of MEN2B patients have mutations in codon 918 (exon 16, tyrosine kinase domain) and rarely in codon 883 of exon 15.

In the case of FMTC, germline mutations are distributed throughout the RET gene with accumulation in exon 13 (codons 768, 790, 791) and exon 14 (codons 804, 844).

Patients with MEN2B associated with codon 918 mutations have a high risk of aggressive MTC at a young age. On the other hand, patients with codon 791 mutations have a relatively low risk of a late onset and slow-growing tumors.

5.6.3. *MEN4*

Given the small number of families and cases with CDKN1B mutations, there are not enough data to suggest a possible genotype–phenotype relationship.

5.6.4. *HPT-JT*

To date, there is no clear genotype–phenotype association, although carriers of CDC73 missense mutations appear to have a higher probability of isolated hyperparathyroidism.

5.7. Penetrance

5.7.1. *MEN1*

Although MEN1 may present any one of the major syndrome constituent manifestations, PHPT is the most common feature and occurs in 95% of MEN1 patients. Pancreatic neuroendocrine tumors occur in 40–75% of MEN1 patients, while PitNETs are identified in 30–55% of patients. Occasionally adrenal cortical carcinoma is reported. Thymic and bronchial carcinoid tumors are present in 2% of MEN1 patients.

5.7.2. *MEN2*

All variants of MEN2 show strong penetrance for MTC; in fact, 90% of MEN2 carriers will develop signs of MTC. MEN2A, which accounts for 75% of MEN2, is characterized by MTC in 90% of adult carriers of deleterious mutations, unilateral or bilateral pheochromocytoma in 50% of cases, and multigland parathyroid tumors in 20–30% of cases.

5.7.3. *MEN4*

Patients with CDKN1B-inactivating pathogenic mutations appear to have a more restricted phenotype, closer to that of MEN1,with a high incidence mainly of PHPT (in 100% of affected subjects) and PitNET (somatotrophic, corticotropic and non-functional adenomas).

5.7.4. *HPT-JT*

CDC73 pathogenic germline mutations generally result in parathyroid adenomas (> 70% of affected individuals), maxillary or mandibular bone fibroids (25–50%), or infrequently, cancers of the parathyroid (15%).

Other manifestations of such CDC73 germline mutations include a high rate of benign and malignant uterine tumors (75% of patients) and renal abnormalities (20%) including cysts, hamartomas and rarely Wilms' tumor.

5.8. Mode of transmission

All of these MEN are usually transmitted by an autosomal dominant mode of transmission. In most cases, the altered gene is inherited from an affected parent (germline mutations).

The remaining cases are the result of new mutations in the gene and occur in patients with no history of the disorder in their family (*de novo* mutations).

5.9. Monitoring

5.9.1. *MEN1*

Recommendations for presymptomatic screening of MEN1 carriers have been established and are based on the youngest age at which manifestations of the disease have been reported in the family. Table 5.1 defines a recommended monitoring model, modified from that described by Thakker and colleagues.

Delays in the diagnosis and/or monitoring of tumors in MEN1 carriers are associated with increased morbidity and mortality.

For first-degree relatives of MEN1 carriers, whose mutational status is unknown, it is recommended that serum prolactin be determined at an annual rate starting at five years of age and serum calcium (corrected for albumin) be determined annually starting at ten years of age.

Manifestations of MEN1	Age at which screening begins	Symptoms	Annual biochemical tests	Imaging
Insulinoma	5 years	Syncope, dizziness, documented hypoglycemia	Insulin and fasting glucose blood level	None
PitNET	5 years[1]	Headaches, visual changes, galactorrhea, growth increase	Prolactin, IGF-1	Brain MRI (every 3 years)
Primary parathyroid/hyperparathyroid adenoma	8 years	Back pain, bone pain, weakness, fatigue, psychiatric changes, kidney stones, nausea, vomiting, constipation; multiple or pathologic fractures	Calcium[2]	None

1 MRI monitoring should begin as soon as the patient is able to tolerate an MRI scan without sedation (usually around the age of five years, but this may vary between individuals).

2 Hypercalcemia at the time of screening should prompt simultaneous assessment of serum calcium and parathyroid hormone (iPTH) to establish a diagnosis of PHPT.

Manifestations of MEN1	Age at which screening begins	Symptoms	Annual biochemical tests	Imaging
Pancreatic NET	10 years	Usually not identified symptomatically; VIPoma can cause profuse diarrhea; glucagonoma associated with hyperglycemia, nausea, polyuria, thirst	Chromogranin A, glucagon, proinsulin, pancreatic polypeptide, vasoactive intestinal polypeptide[3]	Abdominal MRI (annual)
Adrenal adenoma	10 years	None	None	MRI (simultaneous with pancreatic imaging)
Gastrointestinal, bronchial and thymic NET	20 years	Frequently asymptomatic, but history of flushing, diarrhea, wheezing, edema or abdominal pain should raise suspicion	None	CT/MRI chest and abdomen (every 1–2 years)
Gastrinoma (duodenal and pancreatic)	20 years	Abdominal pain, gastric ulcers; use of proton pump inhibitors	Fasting gastrin	None

Table 5.1. *Patient monitoring for MEN1 mutation carriers*

5.9.2. *MEN2*

5.9.2.1. *MTC*

Routine monitoring of MTC includes both serial ultrasound and biochemical monitoring of serum calcitonin levels. Total thyroidectomy, when performed by

3 Pancreatic tumors may not be secretory. Therefore, the additional sensitivity provided by biochemical screening has not been demonstrated.

surgeons experienced in MEN syndromes, is the main preventive strategy to manage the risk of MTC in individuals with pathogenic RET mutations.

DEFINITION.– Thyroidectomy *is the removal of all or part of the thyroid gland. Thyroidectomy is used to treat thyroid disorders such as cancer, non-cancerous enlargement of the thyroid gland (goiter) and overactive thyroid (hyperthyroidism).*

However, genotype and calcitonin levels may also allow the clinician to adjust the age at which thyroidectomy is indicated. For the highest risk allele, p.M918T, thyroidectomy is advised in the first year of life.

For children with high-risk alleles (codons 634 and 883), thyroidectomy may be delayed to balance the risk of surgical complications. These children should have an annual ultrasound and screening for calcitonin levels starting at age three, and thyroidectomy when high levels are detected or no later than age five.

Timing thyroidectomy in individuals with "moderate" risk alleles is very difficult, as this category represents a wide range of penetrance and age of onset associated with different alleles, and considerable variability exists even within families sharing the same mutation.

Therefore, individualization based on specific data and family history can be considered for reasoned surgical planning. Current guidelines for carriers of "moderate" risk alleles recommend thyroidectomy when calcitonin levels show an upward trend or if a biopsy has been performed and shows cytological evidence of MTC in a thyroid lesion.

5.9.2.2. *PHEO*

According to the American Thyroid Association, PHEO screening should begin at 11 years of age for patients with "high" (codons 634 and 883) and "highest" (codon 918) risk alleles, and at 16 years of age for patients with "moderate" risk alleles (all other codons).

Since carriers of pathogenic RET mutations have blood tests for MTC monitoring, blood tests for PHEO (metanephrines and normetanephrines without plasma, or 24-h urine fractionated metanephrines) can be added.

5.9.2.3. *PHPT: hyperparathyroidism*

Screening for PHPT with serum calcium (if normoalbumic) should begin at 11 and 16 years of age for high-risk and moderate-risk allele carriers, respectively. The development of hypercalcemia during monitoring suggests hyperparathyroidism and should be followed by simultaneous measurement of calcium and intact parathyroid hormone (iPTH) while excluding hypovitaminosis D as the cause of PHPT.

5.9.3. *MEN4*

The youngest age (reported in the literature to date) of a patient with CDKN1B disease is 30 years, and they also had acromegaly. Thus, monitoring is primarily clinical and should focus on evidence of excess GH (gigantism/acromegaly) and excess glucocorticoids (Cushing's syndrome).

In children, routine anthropometric evaluation with examination of growth curves is relevant, as PitNETs may exhibit accelerated growth (hypersecretion of GH) or stunted growth with weight gain (hypersecretion of adrenocorticotropic hormone).

Annual blood tests for PHPT (total calcium adjusted for serum albumin) and biochemical monitoring of pituitary secretory somatotrophic adenomas (annual IGF-1) are recommended from adolescence.

5.9.4. *HPT-JT*

Monitoring for carriers of pathogenic germline mutations in CDC73 should begin at five to ten years of age and should include (1) annual biochemical screening for hyperparathyroidism (total calcium, corrected for serum albumin); (2) dental panoramic X-rays every five years; and (3) renal ultrasound every five years.

6

Hereditary Paraganglioma–pheochromocytoma

6.1. Introduction

Paranganglioma (PGL) and pheochromocytoma (PCC) are rare neuroendocrine tumors that tend to occur in the context of genetic predisposition.

PGLs emerge from sympathetic and parasympathetic paraganglions located along the spine from the base of the skull to the pelvis. They may or may not secrete catecholamines. PCCs are generally catecholamine-secreting tumors that develop in the medullary marrow of the adrenal glands. Up to 20% of paragangliomas and PCCs are diagnosed in childhood, the vast majority being PCCs.

NOTE.– The classification of endocrine tumors by the World Health Organization arbitrarily reserves the name PCC for tumors originating from adrenal medullary chromaffin cells, while their extra adrenal counterparts are called paragangliomas.

The autosomal dominant inherited syndromes associated with PCC/PGL include Von Hippel–Lindau syndrome (VHL), multiple endocrine neoplasia type 2 (MEN2), neurofibromatosis type 1 (NF1) and familial hereditary/paragangliomatous disorders (PGL 1–5). The genes involved in these syndromes are VHL, RET, NF1 and succinate dehydrogenase (SDH), respectively. Other susceptibility genes with PCC/PGL-related germline mutations include MAX and TMEM127. Currently, the latter genes do not have specific syndromes related to their mutations.

In this chapter, we will discuss familial hereditary/paragangliomatous disorders (PGL 1–5) due to mutations in the SDHx, SDHF1-2, MAX and TMEM127 genes. The other syndromes (VHL, MEN2 and NF1) are dealt with in specific chapters.

6.2. Prevalence

PCC/PGL have an incidence of two to five cases per million per year. PCCs are rare, with a reported annual incidence of 0.4–9.1 cases per million.

PCCs are usually present in the fourth and fifth decades of life, but can occur at any age. The hereditary form of the disease is more likely to occur in younger patients. Approximately 40% of patients with PCC/PGL have germline mutations in at least one of the 14 susceptibility genes (this number increases to 19 in some literature). The rate of germline mutation in the pediatric population with PCC/PGL is higher, reaching up to 70%.

6.3. When to suspect a PCC/PGL

6.3.1. *Pheochromocytomas*

Most PCC symptoms are related to catecholamine synthesis, as most tumors are functional. The classic triad includes headaches, tachycardia/palpitations and sweating. Although ≤ 25% of patients have the classic triad, about half of them have at least one of the symptoms. Chronic hypertension or episodic and volatile hypertension is the most common symptoms. About 6% of patients experience constipation. Additional paraneoplastic syndromes may also occur, the most common being Cushing's syndrome caused by the ectopic production of adrenocorticotropic hormone.

Polycythemia has been reported due to overproduction or hypersensitization to erythropoietin and is particularly associated with PCCs occurring in the context of mutations in the EPAS1 or EGLN1/2 genes.

DEFINITION.– Polycythemia *is a disease in which there are too many red blood cells in the bone marrow and blood, causing the blood to become more viscous (polycythemia formally exists when the hemoglobin, the number of red blood cells (RBCs) and total RBC volume are all above normal). The number of white blood cells and platelets may also increase.*

Symptoms usually occur simultaneously. However, they are non-specific, raising several diagnostic possibilities. Some patients are asymptomatic, particularly those with small tumors or those who secrete methyl catecholamine metabolites.

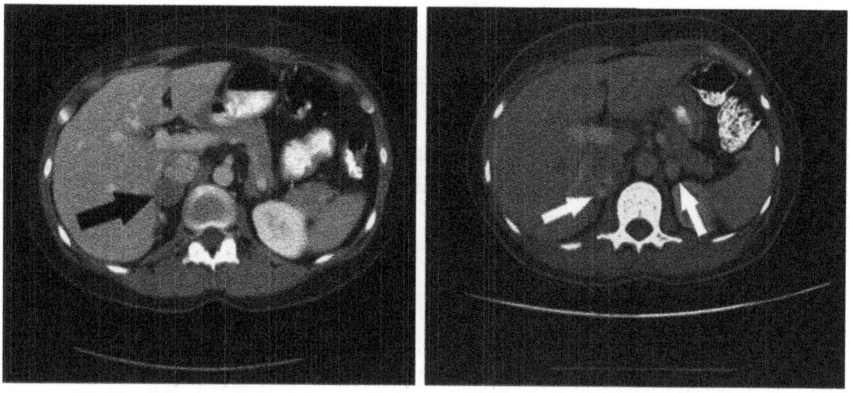

a) b)

Figure 6.1. *Adrenal pheochromocytoma: (a) computed tomography (CT) scan of an adrenal pheochromocytoma (arrow). This tumor produces catecholamines that can cause high blood pressure; (b) CT scan of bilateral pheochromocytomas with contrast products (arrows). This patient has Von Hippel–Lindau syndrome*

6.3.2. *Paragangliomas*

Paragangliomas appear where normal paraganglion cells are present during development or adult life, most often where the cells are most numerous. Paragangliomas at any site may be morphologically identical to PCCs.

6.3.3. *Paragangliomas of the head and neck*

Tumors of the head and neck (HN) account for approximately 20% of all paragangliomas and 0.6% of neoplasms of the HN. The reported incidence ranges from 1/30,000 to 1/100,000. PGLs can occur at any age, starting as young as 13 years of age. The average age is 41 to 47 years with a female–male ratio of up to 8:1.

Hereditary paragagliomas tend to appear in the younger population, about ten years earlier than sporadic forms. They may be associated with paragangliomas or sympathetic PCCs. Paragangliomas of the HN may be bilateral (up to 25%) or multiple (up to 37%), which is common in a hereditary context (up to 80%).

6.3.4. *Sympathetic paragangliomas*

Sympathetic paragangliomas develop at all ages and have an equal distribution among the sexes. The highest incidence is between 40 and 50 years of age. Pediatric paragangliomas are more likely to be bilateral, multifocal and familial. About one third are hereditary and, as with paragangliomas of the HN and PCC, genetic testing should be offered to all patients.

6.4. Tumors

SDHx mutations cause extra adrenal PCC and PGL, including HN PGL. Additional tumors associated with SDHx mutations include renal cell carcinoma (RCC) and gastrointestinal stromal tumors. Renal carcinomas have been reported in patients with SDHB, SDHC and SDHD mutations. Pituitary adenoma and neuroblastoma have also been reported in patients with SDHx mutations.

Familial paraganglioma syndromes have distinct clinical phenotypes depending on the specific SDH mutation.

Due to their rarity, clinical information from patients with mutations in SDHA, SDHC and SDHAF2 is limited.

SDHB, SDHC and SDHD mutations have been reported in patients with the Carney–Stratakis dyad – PCC/PGL and GISTs (gastrointestinal stromal tumors); however, the genetic defect in patients with the Carney triad (PCC/PGL, GIST and pulmonary chondromas) remains unknown.

The clinical features of patients with SDHx germline mutations are summarized in Table 6.1.

Cases of SDHB, SDHC and SDHD germline mutations have been reported in patients with the Carney–Stratakis dyad. GISTs in this dyad are deficient in SDHx. Pediatric patients with PCC and PGL usually have germline mutations of SDHB, SDHD or VHL.

SDHB mutations cause abdominal sympathetic (67%) and thoracic (17.6%) PGL, parasympathetic HN PGL (27.5%) and/or PCC (11.4%). The mean age of presentation is 34 years. Pediatric patients with PCC have an SDHB mutation in 13.6% of cases and the majority of patients develop this tumor at an age of eight years or older.

Disease	Gene	Function	Location	Phenotypic characteristics	Focal: (single or multiple)
Familial hereditary paraganglioma syndrome	SDHx	Succinate dehydrogenase/ mitochondrial complex	/	Pheochromocytoma, paraganglioma	/
PGL1	SDHD	Anchoring subunit	11q23.1	Paraganglioma of the head and neck rarely with abdominal adrenal extraparagangliomas or pheochromocytomas	Multiple
PGL2	SDHAF2	Assembly factor	11q12.2	Paraganglioma of the head and neck	Multiple
PGL3	SDHC	Anchoring subunit	1q23.3	Paraganglioma of the head and neck with rarely abdominal adrenal extraparagangliomas or pheochromocytoma	Multiple
PGL4	SDHB	Catalytic subunit	1p36.13	Extra adrenal paraganglioma, rarely pheochromocytoma or paraganglioma of the head and neck	Multiple
PGL5	SDHA	Catalytic subunit	5p15.33	Extra adrenal pheochromocytoma or paraganglioma	Simple
Hereditary pheochromocytoma	MAX	Transcription factor	14q23.3	Pheochromocytoma	Simple
Hereditary pheochromocytoma	TMEM127	Transmembrane protein involved in mTOR	2q11.2	Pheochromocytoma	Simple

Table 6.1. *Characteristics of hereditary diseases associated with pheochromocytomas and paragangliomas*

Pediatric PCC is associated with SDHD mutations in 6.7% of cases. The mean age of diagnosis of PGL1 is 14 years and the earliest presentation is five years of age. Nonchromaffin cell tumors may also occur in patients with mutated SDHD: clear cell RCC (8%); rare GISTs that are isolated or are part of a Carney–Stratakis dyad or triad; and rare pituitary adenomas.

Solitary PCC: A unilateral PCC is the most common clinical presentation of this tumor. In pediatric patients with a solitary PCC and an associated genetic mutation, VHL accounts for the vast majority of cases, followed by SDHB and SDHD.

SDHA mutations are found in 3% of all PCC/PGL cases. This syndrome has an average age of presentation of 33 years. The youngest reported age is eight years, with only four pediatric cases published to date.

EPAS1 mutations are generally associated with the development of multifocal PGLs. The youngest age reported to date is eight years; although the age of diagnosis of PGL is younger than PCC, PGL can occur simultaneously (33.3%) or after PCC (33.3%) in patients with HIF2A mutations.

TMEM127 mutations have been primarily observed in individuals with PCC, although subsequent studies have shown that carriers of TMEM127 mutations may have extra adrenal PGL, including HN PGL. Bilateral PCCs are common, but the majority of cases are unilateral with a mean age of presentation similar to sporadic tumors (42.8 and 43.2 years, respectively).

MAX mutations appear to be associated with more aggressive disease and were observed primarily in individuals with bilateral PCC or multiple PCC in one adrenal gland (68.4%).

6.5. Genes

Susceptibility genes associated with hereditary PCC/PGL are classified into two groups based on the gene expression profile and the deregulated pathways associated with driver mutations.

6.5.1. *SDHx, SDHAF2 and EPAS1*

Group 1 or pseudo-hypoxia: genes in this group are involved in the oxygen-independent stabilization of hypoxia-inducible factors (HIFs) and activation of downstream oncogenic signaling pathways.

Susceptibility genes in this group include genes involved in the Krebs cycle, such as the four SDH subunits (SDHA-SDHD), SDHAF2 and EPAS1 (codes for a polypeptide designated HIF2A which is a transcription factor) and fumarate hydratase (FH). Mutations in these genes cause an accumulation of intracellular metabolites that inhibit the function of prolyl hydroxylase (PHD2).

These mutations result in a pseudo-hypoxic effect, leading to an aberrant accumulation of HIF. HIF is composed of two subunits, HIF1A and HIF2A. HIF1A interacts with HIF2A via dimerization and acts as a transcription factor for adaptation to hypoxia. When this mechanism is lost due to mutation, angiogenesis occurs.

6.5.2. *TMEM127 and MAX*

Group 2 or kinase signaling pathway: this group comprises the genes associated with the tyrosine kinase receptor and the activation of the downstream signaling pathway. These genes include transmembrane protein 127 (TMEM127) and MYC-associated factor X (MAX).

Activation of tyrosine kinase receptors and downstream signaling pathways, such as PI3K-AKT-mTOR and MYC, affects glycolysis and synthesis of proteins, nucleic acids, amino acids and fatty acids and promotes cell growth.

The MAX gene codes for a protein member of the helix-loop-helix leucine zipperde family, which is therefore a transcription factor and regulates cell proliferation.

6.6. Genotype–phenotype correlations

Although it is well recognized that specific genetic lesions result in different clinical presentations, genotype–phenotype relationships are currently not sufficiently defined.

6.7. Penetrance

SDH mutations are frequently found without a family history, possibly due to low penetrance. In addition, maternal imprinting has been found in patients with mutations in the SDHD and SDHAF2 genes, an epigenetic change that may mask familial inheritance.

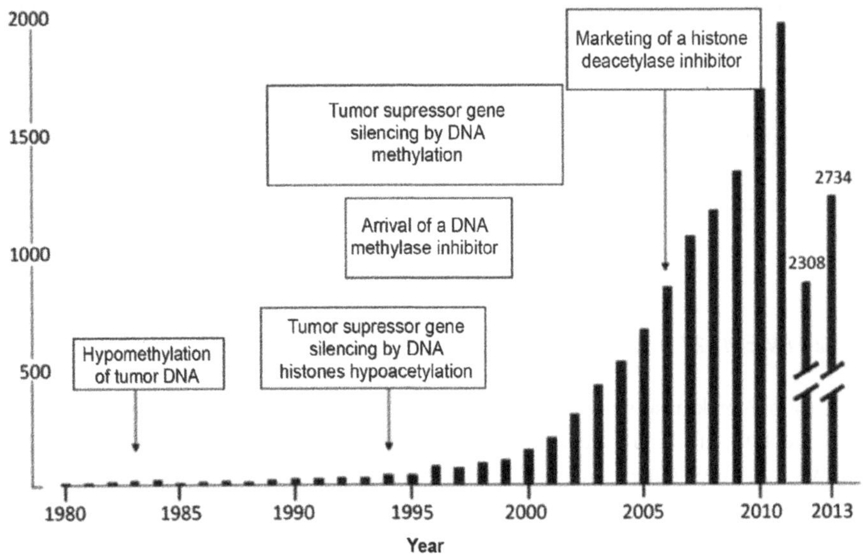

Figure 6.2. *History of publications linking methylation defects to cancer*

COMMENT ON FIGURE 6.2.– *Since the discovery of hypomethylation of tumor DNA in the 1980s, work linking this mechanism to cancers has continued to increase, especially after 2010.*

Mutations in SDHA, SDHAF2 and SDHC are rare and specific penetrance estimates have not been calculated, although some have estimated penetrance of SDHAF2 germline mutations to be 100% at age 45. The penetrance of SDHA mutations is estimated to be low.

For PGL5, which is caused by mutations in the A subunit of the SDH complex, penetrance reaches 38% at age 40.

SDHB mutations cause PGL4 and penetrance reaches 65% at age 40 (some sources give an overall estimate of penetrance of 25–50%). It is estimated that 14% of SDHB carriers develop RCC.

For SDHD germline mutations that predispose carriers to PGL1, the mean age of presentation is 28 years and penetrance exceeds 80% at 40 years of age.

Penetrance of the TMEM127 germline is low; only 20% of patients with TMEM127 germline mutations report a family history of PCC.

For MAX, the overall germline mutation rate is low (1.12%) and penetrance is still unknown at this time.

6.8. Mode of transmission

The predisposition to PCC/PGL, as well as other associated tumors, is either inherited in a strictly autosomal dominant manner (SDHA, SDHB, SDHC and TMEM127) or autosomal dominant manner modified by the parent-of-origin effect. Mutations in SDHD, SDHAF2 and MAX exhibit parent-dependent tumorigenesis, in which tumor formation occurs almost exclusively in the context of paternal transmission of the variant due to maternal imprinting (children inheriting the mutation from their carrier father develop the disease, but children inheriting the mutation from carrier mothers will not).

6.9. Monitoring

Genotype–phenotype relationships are currently not sufficiently defined to justify separate genotype-based monitoring programs.

Monitoring recommendations for PCC/PGL syndromes are similar to those for VHL with respect to PCC/PGL screening (see Table 6.2). However, the existence of silent (non-secretory) paragangliomas, particularly those occurring in the HN – which are more common than in VHL – should be considered, highlighting the importance of radiologic monitoring in PCC/PGL syndrome in addition to biochemical screening. This screening will also facilitate the identification of clear cell RCC, which has rarely been associated with SDHx germline mutations.

Tumor type	Recommended monitoring	Age of screening	Frequency
PCC/PGL	Blood pressure at all medical visits[1]	6–8 years old	Annual (minimum)
	Plasma methoxytyramine	6–8 years old	Annual
	FPM[2, 3, 4, 5] or metanephrines[6] fractionated in urine over 24 h	6–8 years old	Annual
	Optional: serum chromogranin A	6–8 years old	Annual
	Whole body MRI (base of skull to pelvis)[7]	6–8 years old	Biennial
	Optional: contrast MRI of the neck[8]	6–8 years old	Biennial
GIST	Whole blood test (with RBC index)	6–8 years old	Annual

Table 6.2. *Monitoring program. FPM: free plasma metanephrines; RBC: red blood cell*

1 Blood pressure in children should be assessed using age- and height-specific norm ranges.

2 The comparing of values observed in children to pediatric reference intervals for plasma and urine metanephrines should be taken into account.

3 Ideally, to limit false-positive results, FPM should be collected from the patient using an indwelling venous catheter after the patient has been lying on his or her back for 30 min. Clinicians may choose to circumvent this approach, but marginally elevated results should prompt repeat testing under ideal conditions.

4 Many foods and medications can interfere with metanephrine testing and should be avoided prior to testing.

5 Recommended action based on plasma metanephrines: confirm that interfering agents have been avoided prior to testing; if > 4*x* upper limit of the reference range: compatible with disease, proceed with imaging to locate the lesion; if 2*x*–4*x* upper limit of the reference range: repeat testing in two months; if slightly elevated: repeat testing in six months or consider clonidine suppression testing to exclude false positivity.

6 Fractionated metanephrines in 24 h urine are an acceptable alternative to plasma metanephrines once patients are urinary continent.

7 Special attention is also given to the kidneys because of the rare risk of RCC.

8 Depending on the preferences of local radiologists, dedicated MRI of the neck may be preferred to whole body MRI. If this is the case, it should be performed at the same time as whole body MRI.

The sensitivity and specificity of whole body imaging were 87.5% and 94.7%, respectively, while biochemical monitoring gave sensitivity and specificity of 37.5% and 94.5%, respectively.

There are currently no data to support routine imaging for GIST in at-risk patients. No formal studies of the sensitivity of whole body MRI for submucosal gastric masses have been performed, but one would expect the sensitivity to be relatively low for small GISTs.

7

Birt–Hogg–Dubé Syndrome

7.1. Introduction

Birt–Hogg–Dubé (BHD; OMIM #135150) syndrome is due to an alteration in the FLCN gene. It is characterized by variable dermatological stigmas, as well as pulmonary cysts, spontaneous pneumothorax and an increased risk of renal neoplasia.

Skin lesions associated with this condition include fibrofolliculomas, trichodiscomas, perifollicular fibroids and acrochordons. The only cancers associated with BHD syndrome are kidney cancers. However, other tumors have been observed in patients with BHD syndrome.

7.2. Prevalence

The incidence of BHD syndrome is not well known, but is assumed to be underdiagnosed because of the variable penetrance of cutaneous and extra-cutaneous phenotypes. Prevalence is estimated in 1/200,000 births.

7.3. When to suspect BHD syndrome

Fibrofolliculomas are the most common symptoms of BHD syndrome, occurring on the face, neck and upper torso in more than 85% of patients over the age of 25 years. Approximately one quarter of patients with BHD syndrome report a history of spontaneous pneumothorax usually occurring before the age of 40.

In a risk estimate to assess patients with BHD syndrome and their unaffected relatives, BHD patients were seven times more likely to develop renal neoplasia and 50 times more likely to develop spontaneous pneumothorax (age-adjusted) than their unaffected siblings.

DEFINITION.– Pneumothorax *is an abnormal filling of air in the space between the thin layer of tissue covering the lungs and the chest cavity (pleural cavity). This can cause all or part of the lung to collapse.*

Lung involvement in BHD syndrome, in the form of bilaterals, basal and subpleural lung cysts, is observed in more than 80% of cases examined by chest computed tomography (CT).

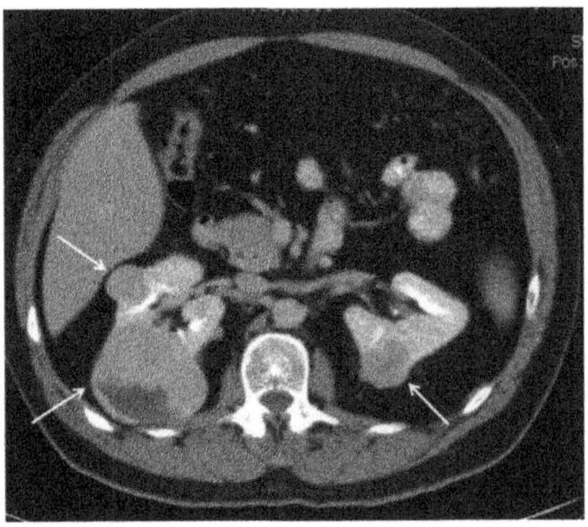

Figure 7.1. *BHD renal tumors, bilateral. Axial view of the mid-section of an individual showing two tumors in the left kidney and one tumor in the right kidney. Renal tumors associated with Birt–Hogg–Dubé are usually multifocal and bilateral. The arrows indicate the locations of the tumors*

7.4. Tumors

Kidney tumors develop in up to one-third of patients with BHD syndrome, at an average age of 50 years. Patients with BHD syndrome most commonly present with renal chromophobic carcinoma (34%) or hybrid oncocytic tumors (50%) with features of chromophobe renal cell carcinoma and renal oncocytoma.

DEFINITION– Oncocytoma *is a benign solid renal tumor consisting primarily or entirely of oncocytes.*

Kidney mass	Frequency (%)	
	General population	Patients with BHD syndrome
Oncocytoma	2–3	5
Chromophobic RCC	< 5	34
Hybrid chromophobic oncocytoma RCC	< 1	50
Clear cell RCC	70–75	9
Papillary RCC	10–15	2

Table 7.1. *Frequency of renal mass type in the general population and in patients with Birt–Hogg–Dubé (BHD) syndrome; RCC = renal cell carcinoma*

Studies have demonstrated a significantly higher risk of developing colon neoplasia in patients with BHD syndrome with the c.1285dupC mutation of the FLCN compared to patients with the c.610delGCinsTA mutation. Other manifestations (i.e. parotid oncocytomas, lipomas, thyroid nodules/cancer, liver cysts) have been reported occasionally in patients with BHD syndrome, but none have been confirmed as part of the clinical picture of this disease.

7.5. Gene

The FLCN tumor suppressor gene encodes a protein called folliculin (FLCN). FLCN has no sequence homology with known functional domains, but X-ray crystallography studies have shown that its C-terminal end shows structural similarity with DENN proteins (differentially expressed in normal cells and neoplasia), which act as guanine nucleotide exchange factors (GEFs) for small Rab GTPases. FLCN forms a complex with the folliculin 1 and 2 interacting proteins (FNIP1, FNIP2) and with the 5' AMP activated protein kinase (AMPK).

Functional studies of FLCN confirm its role in various metabolic pathways and cellular processes including modulation of the mTOR pathway, regulation of biogenesis of PGC1α and mitochondria, cell adhesion and Rho A signaling, control of TFE3/TFEB transcription activity, amino acid–dependent activation of mTORC1 on lysosomes via Rag GTPases and regulation of autophagy.

7.6. Genotype–phenotype correlations

To date, more than 150 different variants of pathogenic FLCN have been reported and deleterious alterations in the gene are found in more than 80% of individuals with BHD syndrome. Genotype–phenotype correlations have been proposed but have not been clearly established.

7.7. Penetrance

Penetrance is usually not complete. Clinical manifestations are very variably expressed by patients with BHD syndrome. These clinical manifestations have varying degrees of penetrance but overall maintain incomplete penetrance.

7.8. Mode of transmission

As with the majority of genetic predispositions to cancer, the mode of transmission of BHD syndrome is autosomal dominant and in most cases the altered gene is inherited from an affected parent (germ mutations). In some individuals, the disorder is due to a spontaneous (*de novo*) genetic mutation that occurs in the egg or sperm of unaffected parents.

7.9. Monitoring

Once a patient is diagnosed with BHD syndrome, an active monitoring program can be initiated based on the individualized presentation. In addition to genetic testing, family members of patients with BHD syndrome may undergo abdominal imaging every 36 months for life.

In general, CT or contrast-enhanced magnetic resonance imaging (MRI) is preferable to ultrasound, as small renal or isoechoic lesions may not be detected by ultrasound. If frequent monitoring examinations are planned, MRI may be preferred over CT to reduce lifetime exposure to radiation.

The general objectives of active monitoring are to detect and treat potentially dangerous injuries and to keep the number of interventions to a minimum. This helps to preserve kidney function and reduce morbidity. If kidney masses are detected, the time intervals for imaging can be modified according to type, size and growth rate. Changing imaging times is particularly important in the presence of clear-cell RCC, since this type of tumor can be more aggressive and associated with a shortened lifespan. Since renal masses greater than 3 cm in diameter have a higher risk of metastasis, intervention should be considered.

Preventive and hygienic measures must be taken to reduce the risk of pneumothorax: air travel is not recommended in the event of a history of recurrent pneumothorax and neither is scuba diving. Cigarettes are also strongly discouraged. It is advisable to be vaccinated against pneumococcus and seasonal flu.

8

RASopathies

8.1. Introduction

RASopathies are a genetically heterogeneous group of disorders caused by germline mutations in genes involved in the RAS-MAPK (mitogen-activated protein kinase) pathway. As a group, RASopathies are one of the largest groups of known malformative syndromes and include neurofibromatosis type 1 (NF1), Legius syndrome, Noonan syndrome, cardiofaciocutaneous syndrome (CFC), capillary malformation/arteriovenous malformation, Noonan syndrome with multiple lentigines (NSML/LEOPARD) and Costello syndrome. RASopathies have many overlapping phenotypic features.

8.2. Prevalence

RASopathies are a group of pathologies which, if considered individually, remain relatively rare. However, if we consider the RASopathies group as a whole (all pathologies including NF1), the prevalence can reach 1/1000 individuals.

8.3. When to suspect RASopathies

The criteria for suspicion of RASopathies are summarized in Table 8.1.

Syndrome	Gene	Clinical phenotype
Neurofibromatosis type 1	NF1	Café au lait spots; intertriginous freckles; neurofibromas and plexiform neurofibromas; Lisch's iris nodules; bone dysplasia; optic glioma; normal or mildly impaired neurocognitive function; predisposition to other cancers

Syndrome	Gene	Clinical phenotype
Noonan syndrome	PTPN11; SOS1; RAF1; KRAS; NRAS; SHOC2; CBL	Characteristics of craniofacial dysmorphic features, including a broad forehead, hypertelorism, downward sloping palpebral fissures, ptosis, high arch palate and low and posteriorly rotating ears; congenital heart defects; small stature; undescended testes; ophthalmological abnormalities; coagulation disorders; normal or mildly impaired neurocognitive function; predisposition to cancer.
Noonan syndrome with multiple lentigines	PTPN11; RAF1	Identical to Noonan syndrome, but with possible development of multiple skin lentigines as individuals get older; uncertain predisposition to cancer.
Capillary malformation-arteriovenous malformation	RASA1	Multifocal capillary malformations that may be associated with arteriovenous malformations and fistulas; uncertain predisposition to cancer.
Costello syndrome	HRAS	Craniofacial features similar to Noonan syndrome, but potentially more pronounced; congenital heart defects; growth delay; short stature; ophthalmologic abnormalities; multiple skin manifestations including papilloma; normal or mildly impaired neurocognitive function; hypotonia; predisposition to cancer.
Cardiofaciocutaneous syndrome	BRAF; MAP2K1; MAP2K2; KRAS	Craniofacial features similar to Noonan syndrome; congenital heart defects; growth delay; short stature; ophthalmologic abnormalities; multiple skin manifestations, including progressive nevus formation; normal or mildly impaired neurocognitive function; hypotonia; uncertain predisposition to cancer.
Legius syndrome	SPRED1	Café au lait spots; intertriginous freckles; macrocephaly; normal or mildly impaired neurocognitive function; no apparent predisposition to cancer.

Table 8.1. *Clinical classification of different types of RASopathies*

8.4. Tumors

The high prevalence of somatic mutations in human RAS genes (KRAS, NRAS and HRAS) and in human BRAF in epithelial cancers of adult solid tumors and melanoma suggests that children with germline mutations in these genes may be predisposed to premature epithelial malignancy or melanoma. In fact, these types of tumors are rare in children with neuro-cardio-facial-cutaneous syndromes, and the most frequently reported types of tumors are myeloid, myogenic and neural tumors. Children with Costello syndrome and Noonan syndrome have the highest incidence of malignancies, with cumulative cancer incidence of 15–20% and 4%, respectively. The most frequently observed tumor types in Costello and Noonan syndromes are rhabdomyosarcoma and neuroblastoma. Bladder cancer of epithelial origin is also observed in adolescents with Costello syndrome. In addition to solid tumors, a myeloproliferative disorder (MPD) is observed in children with Noonan syndrome. In the majority of cases, MPD is transient and benign in nature; however, in some children, it progresses to complete juvenile myelomonocytic leukemia.

8.5. Genes

RASopathies are a class of developmental disorders caused by germline mutations in gene-encoding components or regulators of the RAS/MAPK pathway. The RAS/MAPK pathway is a key signaling pathway that controls cell proliferation, differentiation and survival.

The RAS/MAPK pathway has been extensively studied in the context of ontogenesis, as its somatic deregulation is one of the major causes of cancer. The RAS gene is somatically mutated in approximately 20% of malignancies and BRAF is somatically mutated in approximately 7% of malignancies.

The RAS/MAPK pathway plays a vital role in development and is activated by extracellular signals in the form of growth factors. The RAS genes are a multigenic family consisting of HRAS, NRAS and KRAS. RAS proteins are small GTPases linked to the guanosine nucleotide that function as a critical signaling center in the cell.

To the 17 RASopathies genes already identified (NF1, PTPN11, SOS1, RAF1, KRAS, NRAS, SHOC2, CBL, PTPN11, RAF1, RASA1, HRAS, BRAF, MAP2K1, MAP2K2, KRAS and SPRED1), others have recently been added (RIT1, RRAS, RASA2, A2ML1, SOS2 and LZTR1).

8.6. Genotype–phenotype correlations

With the exception of LEOPARD syndrome (NSML), all mutations identified to date are characterized by an increase in the physiological activity of mutated protein and therefore increased signaling through the RAS/MAPK pathway.

Although the genotype–phenotype relationship is not clear, some authors have proposed the classification of these neuro-cardio-facial-cutaneous syndromes into three groups according to the point at which the RAS/MAPK pathway is affected.

The first group consists of syndromes caused by mutations in the upstream genes, i.e. PTPN11, SOS1 and NF1. In this group, patients tend to have a Noonan-type phenotype, a mild intellectual disability and a greater likelihood of pigmented lesions than ectodermal manifestations. In addition, in the presence of NF1 and PTPN11 mutations, there appears to be a slightly increased risk of leukemia.

The second group includes syndromes caused by mutations in the KRAS gene or downstream. These syndromes mainly affect cognitive functions and the skin, which has redundant folds, keratinization defects and hair anomalies. Although the risk of associated malignancy is low, leukemia can develop.

In the third group are syndromes caused by mutations in HRAS, the main example of which is Costello syndrome. These patients usually have atrial fibrillation (atrial), hyperpigmentation of the skin, papillomatous growths and an increased likelihood of developing soft tissue tumors.

8.7. Penetrance

The disorders have variable expressivity. Some of the genes/mutations do not have complete penetrance.

Penetrance is strong for NSML, it is almost complete for NF1, Noonan syndrome, Legius syndrome and capillary/arteriovenous malformation. Penetrance is complete for Costello syndrome and CFC.

8.8. Mode of transmission

RASopathies are all transmitted in an autosomal dominant manner.

In the case of constitutional mutations, descendants of an affected parent have a 50% probability of inheriting the mutation. However, the situation is more complicated in the case of *de novo* mutations (somatic and/or germinal mosaicism).

8.9. Monitoring

With few exceptions, patients with RASopathies have a slightly increased risk of cancer that warrants greater awareness and rapid assessment when suspicious clinical symptoms are present. Since the risk of childhood cancer is less than 5% in most of these syndromes, routine cancer monitoring is probably not warranted; however, monitoring may be warranted for non-malignant complications.

In patients with CBLS (germline mutations in the CBL gene cause CBL syndrome: CBLS, a variable phenotype characterized by a relatively high frequency of neurological/vascular features, moderate NS features and a high risk of juvenile myelomonocytic leukemia) or with Noonan syndrome (with specific mutations in PTPN11 or KRAS known to be associated with MPD/juvenile myelomonocytic leukemia), an examination every 3–6 months with evaluation of spleen size and differential complete blood count should be considered at birth (or at diagnosis) and should continue until the age of 5.

For most RASopathies, the risk of cancer does not justify routine cancer monitoring. However, exceptions include Costello syndrome, CBL syndrome and Noonan syndrome with specific high-risk mutations. It will be important to assess cancer risks and types of cancer more accurately by enrolling affected individuals in specific monitoring programs.

9

Familial Malignant Melanoma

9.1. Introduction

Melanoma syndromes are separated into two types: "dominant melanoma" and "secondary melanoma". Syndromes in which melanoma is a predominant type of cancer are considered to be dominant melanomas, although other cancers, such as mesothelioma or pancreatic cancer, may also be observed.

These syndromes are associated with defects in CDKN2A, CDK4, BAP1, the microphthalmia-associated transcription factor (MITF) and POT1.

Secondary melanoma syndromes have an increased risk of melanoma, but less than other cancers in the syndrome, such as breast and ovarian cancer syndrome, Cowden syndrome, *xeroderma pigmentosum*, familial retinoblastoma, Muir–Torre syndrome (MTS) and Li–Fraumeni syndrome.

DEFINITION.– Retinoblastoma *is a tumor that forms in the tissues of the retina (layers of light-sensitive nerve tissue at the back of the eye). Retinoblastoma usually occurs in children under 5 years of age. It can be hereditary or non-hereditary (sporadic).*

Melanomas have also been observed in families generally prone to particular types of malignancies, such as the familial atypical multiple mole melanoma (FAMMM) syndrome and its variant melanoma-astrocytoma syndrome (MAS).

Germline mutations in cyclin-dependent kinase inhibitor 2A (CDKN2A or p16) and, less frequently, mutations in cyclin-dependent kinase 4 (CDK4) are the most commonly identified genetic abnormalities in these families.

An important overlap, previously unknown, has been identified: melanoma predisposing genes may be associated with other types of cancer and other genes predisposing to different cancers may increase the risk of melanoma.

Finally, international whole genome association studies (GWAS) have led to the discovery of at least 20 common susceptibility loci associated with reproducible skin melanoma, which will not be discussed here.

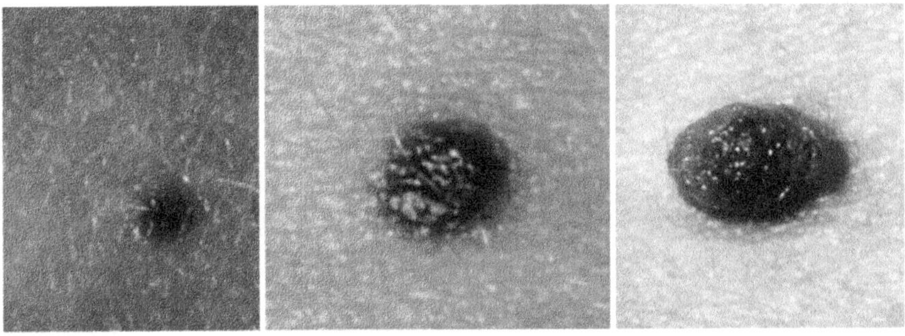

a) b) c)

Figure 9.1. *Beauty spots*

COMMENT ON FIGURE 9.1.– *A mole is a growth on the skin that develops when pigment cells (melanocytes) multiply in clusters. Most adults have between 10 and 40 common moles. Another name for a mole is nevus and the plural is nevi.*

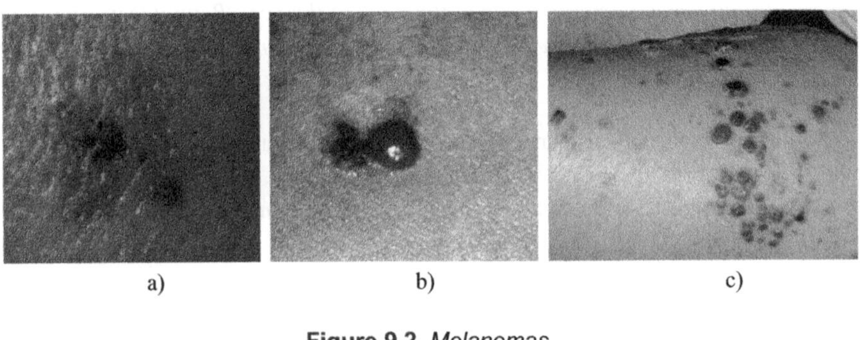

a) b) c)

Figure 9.2. *Melanomas*

COMMENT ON FIGURE 9.2.– *(a) Melanoma in situ: a dark pigmented central lesion surrounded by an ill-defined area of lighter beige pigmentation; this melanoma in situ represents a malignant melanocytic process that has not yet invaded the dermis; (b) advanced malignant melanoma: on the left is a superficial melanoma blemish with early radial spread, on the right and contiguous to the blemish is a pink (amelanotic) nodule of melanoma in a deeply invasive vertical growth phase; (c) metastatic melanoma: numerous pink/purple nodules and eroded blemishes are present on the proximal thigh.*

9.2. Prevalence

Up to 40% of families with recurrent melanomas have a CDKN2A germline mutation, whereas CDK4 mutations are rarely detected in familial melanomas.

The prevalence of CDKN2A mutations was found to be heterogeneously distributed among melanoma patients in different geographic areas.

In fact, a latitude incidence gradient has been described in detail: the highest incidence rates are found in the populations of Australia and New Zealand, followed by the United States and Scandinavian and Central European countries, while in Black African, Asian and South American populations the incidence rate is considerably lower.

It has been estimated that BAP1 mutations are present in approximately 22% of families with familial uveal melanoma, compared to 2–4% in families with uveal melanoma not selected on this basis.

9.3. When to suspect familial malignant melanoma

Familial aggregation of the disease is considered to be responsible for the presence of a transmitted genetic mutation. However, true hereditary melanomas (i.e. transmission through a single multi-generational unilateral parental branch, multiple primary lesions and early onset of the disease) are uncommon.

Since there are several types of cancers that can be associated with melanoma, all of these types of cancers count as indications for genetic testing (see Table 9.1).

Type of cancer	Criteria	Points per occurrence
Melanoma	Occurrence in the index case with melanoma or in a relative of the first or second degree[1]	1 or 1.5
Astrocytoma[2]	Occurrence in the index case with melanoma or in a relative of the first or second degree	1.5
Breast	Occurrence in index, first- or second-degree relative under 45 years of age	1
	Occurrence of bilateral or triple negative breast cancer in the index case in a first- or second-degree relative	1
	Occurrence in a man	1
Colon	Occurrence in the index case or a first-degree relative under 50 years of age	1
	Index cases with more than five adenomatous polyps occurring at less than 50 years of age	1
Ovary	Occurrence in the index case or in a relative of the first or second degree	1
Pancreas[3]	Occurrence in the index case or in a relative of the first or second degree	1.5
Prostate	The index case has had metastatic prostate cancer and/or a Gleason score greater than 7 at diagnosis	1[3]
High frequency	Occurrence in the index case (with melanoma) of two or more first- or second-degree related breast, colon or prostate cancers that do not meet the above criteria	1
BAP1 syndrome	Occurrence in the index case or a first-degree relative of uveal melanoma, paraganglioma, mesothelioma, atypical Spitz tumors or clear cell renal carcinoma	1.5 per cancer type
Perform genetic testing if the score is 3 points or more		

Table 9.1. *Assessment tool for genetic testing (in the context of suspicions of melanoma syndrome)*

1 First-degree relatives include parents, siblings and children; second-degree relatives are blood relatives that include grandparents, grandchildren, aunts, uncles, nephews, nieces or half-brothers and half-sisters.

2 Pancreatic cancer and astrocytoma score 1.5 due to the increased incidence of dominant melanoma syndromes caused by a CDKN2A mutation.

3 The criteria listed suggest a hereditary pattern that may meet the standard criteria for monogenic or cancer-specific panels without association with melanoma. Any individual or family with these results should be considered for genetic testing regardless of their melanoma status. However, if the criteria are met in the context of melanoma, genes that may be associated with melanoma should be tested in addition.

COMMENT ON TABLE 9.1.– *For points per occurrence: 1 point in geographical zones with moderate or high incidence of melanoma and 1.5 points in geographical zones with low incidence. Zones with an age-standardized incidence rate of < 10 per 100,000 population are considered low incidence zones.*

DEFINITION.– Spitz's tumor *(or Spitz's nevus) is a rare melanocytic lesion composed of large epithelioid and/or spindle-shaped cells. It usually presents in childhood or adolescence as a strongly circumscribed, dome-shaped, pinkish-red papule or blemish, usually located on the face or lower extremities.*

9.4. Tumors

9.4.1. *CDKN2A*

Families carrying a pathogenic mutation in CDKN2A have an increased risk of melanoma, pancreatic cancer and possibly neurological tumors such as astrocytoma. Individuals from these families often, but not always, have a large number of atypical moles. A substantially increased number of atypical moles in the context of a CDKN2A mutation has been called FAMMM syndrome, although it is also called familial melanoma and pancreatic cancer (FMPC) syndrome, because of the increased risk of pancreatic cancer.

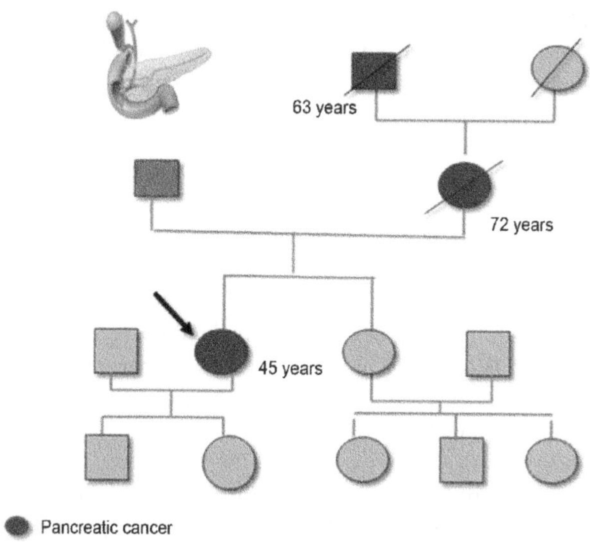

Figure 9.3. *Pancreatic cancer in the context of family aggregation*

While some families with CDKN2A germline mutations are prone to the development of melanomas only, other families develop melanomas, astrocytomas and occasionally other neoplasms of the nervous system, including tumors of the peripheral nerve sheath and meningiomas.

9.4.2. *BAP1*

BAP1 has been identified as the gene causing predisposition to tumors including atypical Spitz tumors, cutaneous and uveal melanomas, mesotheliomas and clear cell renal carcinomas. Cutaneous and uveal melanomas are present in only about 30% and 13% of BAP1 mutation carriers reported to date, respectively.

9.4.3. *MITF*

The rare germline mutation of MITF E318K has been associated with multiple primary melanomas, nodular melanoma and/or renal cell carcinoma (RCC) and may thus play a role in the aggressive, fast-growing form of the disease.

9.4.4. *POT1*

Recently, POT1 mutations have been described not only in families with multiple melanomas, but also in families with predominantly chronic lymphocytic leukemia, predominant glioblastoma, predominant thyroid cancer or families with Li–Fraumeni-like syndrome.

9.5. Genes

9.5.1. *CDKN2A*

The CDKN2A gene locus codes for two melanoma predisposition genes with different functions: CDKN2A/p16, a tumor suppressor that imposes control through the retinoblastoma (Rb) pathway, and CDKN2A/ARF, another tumor suppressor with a function in the p53 pathway.

Although CDKN2A/p16 is the most common and best characterized dominant melanoma predisposition gene, several other less common predisposition genes are associated with an inherited risk of melanoma and other cancers, including alternative transcriptase of CDKN2A (CDKN2A/ARF), CDK4, telomerase reverse transcriptase (TERT), protection of telomeres 1 (POT1), adrenocortical dysplasia (ACD), telomeric repeat binding factor-2 (TERF2), TERF2-interacting protein (TERF2IP), BRCA1-associated protein 1 (BAP1) and MITF.

DEFINITION.– Microphthalmia *is a severe developmental disorder of the eye in which one or both eyes are abnormally small and have anatomical malformations.*

9.5.2. *MITF*

MITF is a transcription factor acting as a master gene for the homeostasis of melanocytes. Deleterious mutations interfere with the SUMOylation of MITF, resulting in increased MITF transcription activity, thereby enhancing the oncogenic role of MITF and reducing the senescence program, potentially promoting melanoma progression *in vivo*.

9.5.3. *POT1*

Like ACD and TERT, POT1 is a gene associated with telomere maintenance. POT1 is associated with the telomeres Shelterin complex, which regulates telomere protection and telomerase accessibility.

9.6. Genotype–phenotype correlations

The tumor spectrum reported in the family history is distinct between those who have BAP1 germline mutations and those who do not. Specifically, families without BAP1 mutations have lower rates of malignant mesothelioma (MMe) and RCC than those with BAP1 mutations.

Although no clear association between genotype and phenotype has been identified in BAP1 syndrome, it appears that almost all patients who develop mesothelioma tend to carry truncated germline mutations in the BAP1 gene.

9.7. Penetrance

High-penetrance germline mutations in CDKN2A, CDK4, BAP1, MITF, TERT, POT1, ACD, TERF2IP and POLE appear to contribute to the development of cutaneous melanomas (CM) in certain families with a high recurrence of melanomas among its members.

The CDKN2A gene locus is involved in about 20–40% of large high-risk families. Patients with CDKN2A mutations have a lifetime risk of developing melanoma of 60–90%.

The very fair skin phototype (RHC: Red Hair Color, associated with fair skin) and the presence of MCR1 variants considerably increase the penetrance of pathogenic CDKN2A mutations. The penetrance of the CDKN2A mutation (in terms of the risk of developing cutaneous melanoma) appears to be higher in women.

CDK4 is a less frequently observed gene that confers a lifetime risk of melanoma of about 70%.

MITF has been identified as a medium-penetrance melanoma susceptibility gene. The low-penetrance variant in MITF (p.E318K) has been shown to increase the risk of melanoma (twofold) as well as the risk of developing RCC.

9.8. Mode of transmission

Autosomal dominant transmission applies to all the melanoma predisposition genes discussed in this chapter (CDKN2A, CDK4, POT1, BAP1 and MITF).

9.9. Monitoring

In melanoma-dominant or melanoma-subordinate families or in individuals with a BAP1, CDK4, CDKN2A, MITF or POT1 mutation, individuals should be informed of the importance of prevention and early detection of melanoma. These individuals should receive education on photoprotection and monthly skin self-examination as well as regular skin screening by a health care professional.

The frequency of examinations by a health care provider should be adapted according to the risk of developing melanoma and the difficulty of performing the examination. High-risk subjects should be examined more frequently, every 3–12 months.

Melanoma syndromes have also been associated with uveal melanomas, RCCs, astrocytomas and other neurological cancers, mesotheliomas and paragangliomas. Any family which carries a mutation in the susceptibility genes for syndromes that include these different types of cancers, or which has these types of cancers reported in its members, should be carefully monitored for early signs and symptoms of these cancers. For example, ophthalmologic examinations should be performed every

6–12 months in BAP1 mutation carriers. Carriers of the BAP1 mutation should also be explicitly warned of asbestos exposures, given their predisposition to mesothelioma. An annual screening MRI may be warranted if the family history or causal mutation is associated with multiple internal malignancies.

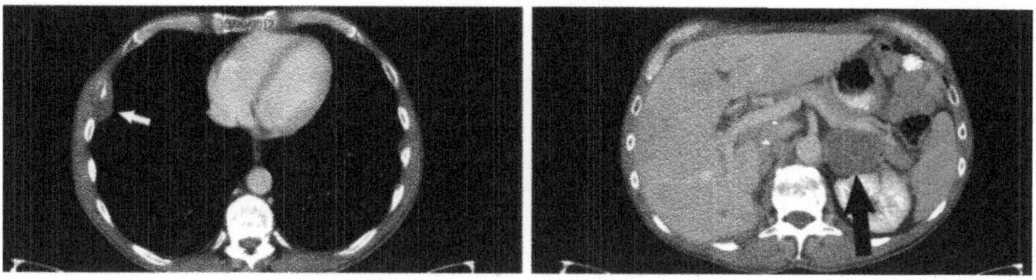

a) b)

Figure 9.4. *Metastatic melanoma: (a) computed tomography (CT) scan of the rib, showing metastases of the melanoma (arrow); (b) CT scan of the adrenals showing metastases of the melanoma (arrow)*

10

Gorlin Syndrome

10.1. Introduction

Nevoid basal cell carcinoma (BCC) syndrome, also known as Gorlin syndrome (GS), is caused by aberrant activation of the hedgehog (Hh) sonic pathway. The presence of multiple BCCs, odontogenic jaw keratocysts, palmar or plantar fossae, falx cerebri calcification, bifid ribs, and a family history of BCC are characteristic of this syndrome.

GS is due to mutations in the PTCH1 gene (transmembrane protein patched homolog 1) in the majority of cases observed. However, in rare cases mutations of the SUFU (suppressor of fused) gene and the PTCH2 gene (in very rare cases) are reported in patients suffering from GS.

10.2. Prevalence

GS is a rare disease and its prevalence has so far not been accurately estimated. The different estimates range from about 1/57,000 to 1/164,000 individuals. The prevalence is the same in men and women (no gender difference).

10.3. When to suspect GS

In addition to the major characteristics cited in the introduction, many minor criteria have been described. A diagnosis of GS requires the presence of at least two major characteristics or the presence of one major characteristic and two minor characteristics.

Major criteria
I. Multiple basal cell carcinoma (BCC) less than 20 years old, or more than 10 basal cell nevi.
II. Any histological odontogenic keratocyst observed on the panoramic radiograph as a zone of translucency or a polyostotic bone cyst.
III. Palmar or plantar fossae (three or more).
IV. Ectopic calcification: lamellar (leaf) calcification of falx or evidence of early calcification in an individual under 20 years of age.
V. First-degree relative with multiple BCCs.
Minor criteria
I. Congenital skeletal abnormality: bifid, jowls or missing ribs, or bifid, wedged or fused vertebrae.
II. Occipital-frontal circumference > 97 percentile (macrocephaly), with frontal lobe.
III. Cardiac or ovarian fibroids.
IV. Medulloblastoma in children (primary neuroectodermal tumor).
V. Lymphomasenteric or pleural cysts.
VI. Congenital malformation: cleft lip and/or palate, polydactyly.
VII. Ocular abnormality (strabismus, hypertelorism, congenital cataracts, coloboma, microphtalmia).

Table 10.1. *Diagnostic criteria for Gorlin syndrome*

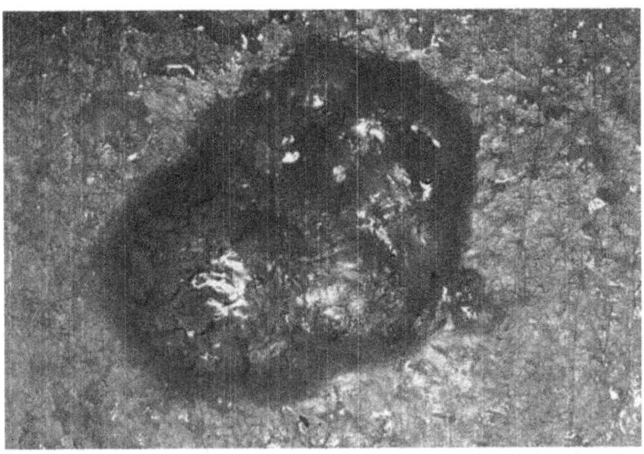

Figure 10.1. *Photograph of basal cell carcinoma*

10.4. Tumors

The most common feature of this syndrome is the development of BCCs during puberty, which are often more clinically aggressive than those seen in the general population. Many patients, particularly those with higher UV exposure or fairer skin, can develop hundreds of BCCs over the course of their lives. BCC development occurs most frequently on the face, followed by the trunk and limbs. GS patients also develop other neoplasms, such as desmoplastic medulloblastoma, meningioma, rhabdomyosarcoma, ovarian and cardiac fibroids, and mesenteric keratocysts.

10.5. Genes

The PTCH1 (patched 1) gene codes for a transmembrane receptor found in early stages of the so-called Hh signaling pathway. The function of PTCH1 is the suppression of the SMO (smoothened) gene. In vertebrates, intracellular signaling activity is mediated by GLI zinc finger transcription factors. It has been shown that suppression of SMO leads to the formation of GLI repressors blocking GLI translocation in the nucleus.

In the normal case of the Hh signaling pathway, the binding of PTCH1 to the Hh ligands results in the release of SMO (SMO is no longer suppressed by PTCH1). Activation of SMO prevents the SUFU gene from inhibiting GLI transcription factors. Overactivation of GLI transcription factors promotes uncontrolled cell growth and cancer.

Mutations in the PTCH1 gene that result in functional loss of the PTCH1 protein result in constitutive activation of the Hh and GS signaling pathway. Similarly, in rare cases, inactivating mutations in the SUFU gene also lead to constitutive activation of the Hh pathway and may also cause GS.

10.6. Genotype–phenotype correlations

Families with identified mutations in one of the susceptibility genes tend to be diagnosed earlier and develop more jaw cysts and bifid ribs, or a skeletal abnormality than families where no mutation has been identified. Patients with a missense variant in PTCH1 are diagnosed later and are less likely to develop at least 10 BCCs and jaw cysts than those with other types of pathogenic PTCH1 mutations. Patients with SUFU pathogenic variants are significantly more likely than those with PTCH1 pathogenic variants to develop medulloblastoma, meningioma or ovarian fibroma but less likely to develop jaw cysts.

10.7. Penetrance

Mutations in PTCH1 are found in 40–85% of patients meeting the diagnostic criteria for GS. Penetrance is nearly complete, but phenotypic expression is variable and does not correlate with the type of PTCH1 mutation.

10.8. Mode of transmission

As with most genetic predispositions to cancer, the mode of transmission of GS is the autosomal dominant mode. In most cases, the altered gene is inherited from an affected parent (germ mutations). The remaining cases are the result of new mutations in the gene and occur in patients with no history of the disorder in their family (*de novo* mutations).

10.9. Monitoring

The management of patients with GS requires a multidisciplinary approach. Screening for non-cutaneous lesions in GS involves radiological monitoring, including cerebral MRI every year for up to eight years, digital panoramic (panorex) X-ray of the jaw every year until the first jaw cyst develops, cardiac ultrasound, spinal X-ray and pelvic ultrasound (in women). Although difficult to avoid, exposure to ionizing radiation should be minimized. Additional recommendations include developmental, cognitive, ophthalmologic and psychological assessments to establish a course of action.

Prevention of exposure to UV radiation and frequent scans from an early age reduce the risk of developing BCC. Therefore, DNA-based tests for diagnosis purposes could be beneficial for young children with unclear clinical features.

Guidelines for monitoring carriers of mutations in susceptibility genes have been established and include cerebral magnetic resonance imaging once a year for 1–7 years, neurological examinations twice a year, pantomograms every 12–18 months starting at eight years of age, annual dermatological examinations and cardiological examinations according to signs and symptoms.

PART 2

Infracentesimal Syndromes

11

Li–Fraumeni Syndrome

11.1. Introduction

Li–Fraumeni syndrome (LFS) is a rare cancer-predisposing condition caused by germline mutations in TP53, the gene encoding the transcription factor TP53.

LFS is characterized by the development of a broad spectrum of malignant tumors in children and adults, including six common "major" cancers: soft tissue sarcomas (STS), osteosarcoma (OS), pre-menopausal breast cancer, central nervous system (CNS) tumors, adrenal cortical carcinoma (ACC) and leukemia (including lymphoid and myeloid leukemia, myelodysplastic syndrome and, to a lesser extent, lymphoma).

DEFINITION.– Lymphoma *is a cancer that starts in the cells of the immune system. There are two types of lymphomas. Hodgkin's lymphoma is marked by the presence of a type of cells called Reed–Sternberg cells. Non-Hodgkin's lymphomas include a large and diverse group of cancers of cells of the immune system. Non-Hodgkin's lymphomas can be divided into cancers that have an indolent (slow-growing) and aggressive (fast-growing) course. These subtypes behave and respond differently to treatment. Hodgkin's and non-Hodgkin's lymphomas can occur in both children and adults, and the prognosis and treatment depend on the stage and type of cancer.*

DEFINITION.– Osteosarcoma *is a bone cancer that usually affects the large bones of the arm or leg. Also known as osteogenic sarcoma, it occurs most often in young people and affects more men than women.*

Constitutional Oncogenetics,
Noureddine BOUKHATEM. © ISTE Ltd 2021.

11.2. Gene

TP53 is located on chromosome 17p13.1 and covers approximately 20 kb of genomic DNA. It is composed of 14 exons of which 10 exons code for the TP53 protein of 393 full-length amino acids, one non-coding exon (exon 1) and three alternative exons (exons 2/3, 9b, 9c).

In non-stressed cells, TP53 levels are kept low via a negative regulatory feedback mechanism mediated by MDM2 (E3 ubiquitin ligase mouse double minute 2 homolog), whose expression is induced by TP53.

Following exposure to genotoxic stressors such as ionizing radiation, oxidative stress and nucleotide depletion, TP53 and MDM2 proteins become phosphorylated. As a result, the MDM2–TP53 interaction is weakened. This weakening reduces TP53 degradation, allowing TP53 to accumulate, associate and bind to specific DNA sequences. Functional TP53 tetramers then induce the expression of numerous downstream target genes that regulate critical cellular processes such as cell cycle arrest, apoptosis and DNA repair.

11.3. Tumors

The risk that carriers of the TP53 germline mutation develop one or more neoplasms is estimated to be 50% at the age of 30–31 years for women and 46 years for men. This risk approaches 70–100% at age 70 for both sexes.

Breast cancer is the most common risk and accounts for about 25–30% of all cancers in LFS families. In contrast to the BRCA1/2 mutation situation, breast cancer appears to occur exclusively (there is no predisposition to ovarian cancer) in women with LFS. In women with apparently sporadic breast cancer at an age younger than 30 years, 3–8% of women with apparently sporadic breast cancer have a germline TP53 mutation.

Together, STS and OSs account for 25–38% of LFS-related malignancies and are the most common cancers in children and adolescents. The prevalence of STS is estimated to range from 17.8–27%, while the prevalence of OS ranges from 13.4–16%. Rhabdomyosarcoma (RMS) often occurs before the age of five and OS before the age of 30.

Tumors of the CNS account for 9–14% of LFS tumors, the most common type being glioblastoma/astrocytoma. Medulloblastomas, ependymomas, supratentorial primary neuroectodermal tumors and choroid plexus carcinomas have also been reported. The age of onset of CNS cancers is biphasic, with a first peak in childhood and a second peak between 20 and 40 years of age (median 16 years).

Adrenocortical carcinoma develops in 6–13% of LFS patients, with a bimodal age distribution peaking before the age of five years and again between the fourth and fifth decades of life.

Leukemias, including acute lymphoblastic leukemia (ALL), acute myeloid leukemia (AML) and myelo dysplastic syndrome (MDS), have a prevalence of 2–4% in carriers of the TP53 germline mutation. The prevalence of leukemia is estimated to be between 2–4%. Lymphoma is somewhat less common, with a prevalence of 2%. The median age of onset of leukemia is 12 years (extremes being 2–35 years) and 13 years (extremes being 2–42 years) for lymphomas.

In addition to the primary cancers, patients with LFS develop additional malignant tumors, many of which occur at earlier ages, including colorectal, pulmonary, pancreatic, melanoma, prostate, renal, testicular, laryngeal, cervico-cervical and ovarian cancers.

11.4. Genetics

The mode of transmission of LFS is autosomal dominant. The distribution of TP53 germline mutations in LFS is similar to that of somatic mutations identified in tumors, with the majority clustering in the DNA-binding domain where there are six recurrent mutations involving codons 175 (R175H), 245 (G245S), 248 (R248Q, R248W), 273 (R273H), and 282 (R282W). Mutations in intronic or regulatory regions are also reported; however, their functional significance remains to be elucidated.

Families with missense mutations within the TP53 DNA-binding domain have a more strongly penetrating phenotype than families with other mutations (nonsense or truncating) or no identified mutations. More recently, a significantly earlier onset of tumors was observed in patients with missense mutations (mean tumor age 23.8 years) compared to those with deletions/insertions with or without reading frame shifts, nonsense mutations and genomic rearrangements (28.5 years).

ACC appears to be the only type among LFS-associated cancers that is consistently linked to germline mutations occurring outside the DNA binding domain of the TP53 gene.

11.5. Monitoring

For individuals of childbearing age, genetic counseling should be offered to discuss the risks of recurrence. Parents with a TP53 germline mutation may consider prenatal testing, as well as preimplantation genetic diagnosis.

The objectives of cancer monitoring are to improve patient management by enabling early detection and treatment of tumors. In general, monitoring is best suited to solid neoplasms, where the prognosis may be better after complete resection of the presented tumor.

Total body magnetic resonance imaging has been shown to be feasible for pediatric cancer screening and is advantageous because of its ability to quickly scan multiple body parts and avoid ionizing radiation. However, a high rate of incidental findings requiring follow-up imaging examinations, and in some cases biopsy of suspicious lesions and high rates of false positives, are major drawbacks.

Small tumors that are completely resected may require little or no chemotherapy or radiation therapy. In theory, this could minimize the risk of secondary cancers associated with treatment. Although the diversity of cancer types and their age of onset make screening in LFS difficult, a feasible multimodal screening protocol (the Toronto protocol: using physical examination in conjunction with frequent blood tests and imaging) has recently been developed and has been associated with a significant improvement in survival in individuals with LFS.

12

Ataxia–telangiectasia

12.1. Introduction

Ataxia–telangiectasia (A–T) is a widely documented genomic instability syndrome. A–T leads to neurodegeneration (mainly cerebellar atrophy), immunodeficiency, oculocutaneous telangiectasia (dilated blood vessels), severely reduced thymus and gonad sizes, endocrine abnormalities, a predisposition to cancer and variable susceptibility to DNA-damaging agents, especially those that induce double-stranded DNA breaks (DSBs).

The main cause of all variants of the disease is mutations in the autosomal ATM (A–T mutated) gene.

12.2. Gene

ATM (A–T mutated) is located at 11q22-23 and codes for the protein ATM, a multifunctional protein kinase. The ATM gene spans 184 kb and contains 66 exons producing 13 kb mRNA. It is extremely rich in sequence variation.

ATM is a homeostatic protein kinase that plays a very wide range of roles in various cellular circuits. ATM is a member of the PI-3 kinase-like protein kinases (PIKK). This family also contains the mTOR protein, which regulates many signaling pathways based on nutrient levels, growth factors and energy balance.

The most widely documented function of ATM, and the one associated with its most vigorous activation, is the mobilization of the complex signaling network that responds to DSBs. ATM supports other DNA repair pathways that respond to a variety of genotoxic stresses, including single-strand break repair (SSBR).

Constitutional Oncogenetics,

12.3. Tumors

Patients affected by A–T are more prone to lymphoid malignancies in childhood, but they are also at risk of developing epithelial cancers later in life. Cancers of the breast, lung, digestive and genitourinary tract, brain and parotid have been described, but their incidence remains poorly understood.

12.4 Genetics

ATM is associated with an autosomal recessive transmission mode. Patients with the severe form of A–T are homozygous or heterozygous for the null ATM alleles. The incidence is between 1/40,000 and 1/200,000 live births in different human populations.

The corresponding mutations generally lead to the truncation of the ATM protein and subsequently to its loss due to the instability of the truncated derivatives; a smaller proportion of the mutations create amino acid substitutions that suppress the catalytic activity of ATM.

On the other hand, heterozygosity for a pathogenic variant of ATM is present in 1–2% of the adult population. These individuals are phenotypically normal, but their risk of breast cancer is about two to three times higher than that of the general population.

12.5. Monitoring

Since the interpretation of ATM heterozygosity can be difficult, with more than 170 variants of missense and numerous truncating mutations, genetic counseling for women with pathogenic ATM variants is recommended for them to set up appropriate monitoring.

With the possible exception of the V2424G variant, which could be considered a high-risk gene variant, ATM is considered to confer a moderate lifetime risk of breast cancer.

Annual mammography and magnetic resonance imaging (MRI), in addition to routine breast examination, for a pathogenic variant of ATM in heterozygous women "with a clear family history" of breast cancer are recommended.

Patients with A–T syndrome are sensitive to the effects of ionizing radiation. However, the evidence for radiation therapy in carriers of pathogenic variant ATM is mixed: some data suggest increased toxicity, others suggest an improved clinical benefit. ATM status should therefore not be used to make therapeutic decisions in radiotherapy.

13

Hyperparathyroidism

13.1. Introduction

Inherited forms of primary hyperparathyroidism (PHPT) are a clinically and genetically heterogeneous group of diseases, accounting for approximately 10–15% of PHTP cases. They may occur in syndromes (multiple endocrine neoplasia syndromes (MEN1, MEN2A, MEN4); hyperparathyroidism jaw tumor (HPT-JT) syndrome) that have been discussed in Chapter 5 (endocrine neoplasia) or in non-syndromic forms (familial isolated hyperparathyroidism (FIHPT), familial hypocalciuric hypercalcemia (FHH) and neonatal severe hyperparathyroidism (NSHPT)), which are treated here. The term FIHPT is applied to a subgroup of patients with a family history of autosomal dominant PHPT without evidence of other endocrinopathies.

FHH1-3 are autosomal dominant diseases with a high degree of variable penetrance and expressivity. The type 1 variant, which accounts for approximately 65% of all FHH cases, results from a mutation by loss of heterozygous gene function (CASR: calcium-sensing receptor; chromosome 3q21.1). FHH type 2 is caused by mutations in the gene (GNA11: guanine nucleotide binding protein, alpha-11; chromosome 19p13.3). FHH type 3 is associated with missense gene mutations (AP2S1: adaptor-related protein complex 2, sigma-1 subunit; chromosome 19q13.3).

NSHPT is most often caused by a homozygous loss of function of the CASR gene.

13.2. Gene

GCM (glial cell missing; chromosome 6p24.2) encodes a 506 amino acid transcription factor that is necessary for parathyroid development and is expressed in the parathyroid glands of developing and adult individuals.

Recent studies indicate that glial cell missing 2 (GCM2) is a parathyroid proto-oncogene and that activating germline mutations in the C-terminally conserved inhibitory domain of GCM2 can cause FIHPT.

The protein coded by AP2S1 (adaptor related protein complex 2 subunit sigma 1) is implicated in many pathways. Among its related pathways are regulation of activated PAK-2p34 by proteasome-mediated degradation and lipoprotein metabolism.

The GNA11 gene codes for one component, the alpha (α) subunit (G_{11}), of a protein complex called a guanine nucleotide-binding protein (G protein). The G11 protein plays many roles in cells. It interacts with another protein called the calcium-sensing receptor (CaSR) to affect processes that regulate calcium levels in the blood.

The CASR gene codes for a protein covering 1,078 amino acids that detects extracellular calcium levels.

13.3. Tumors

13.3.1. *FIHPT*

In most cases, the resected parathyroid glands show signs of single or multiple parathyroid adenomas or hyperplasia of the main cells. The increased incidence of parathyroid carcinoma in some families most likely reflects the inclusion of patients with CDC73 mutations.

13.3.2. *FHH*

FHH is usually asymptomatic, however adults with FHH may rarely have recurrent inflammation of the pancreas (pancreatitis), an accumulation of calcium crystals in certain joints of the body (chondrocalcinosis) and an accumulation of calcium in the veins (vascular calcification). There is a risk of developing a localized parathyroid adenoma, but this risk is very rare.

13.3.3. *NSHPT*

In general, the parathyroid glands are strongly and symmetrically enlarged, with histological evidence of diffuse hyperplasia of the main cells. Clonality studies have shown that parathyroid proliferation in this disorder represents polyclonal processes.

13.4. Genetics

13.4.1. *FIHPT*

A variety of mutations have been reported in patients with suspected FIHPT, including those associated with MEN1 (0–23%), CASR (14%) and CDC73 (rare). Recent studies have implicated the gene (GCM2glial cell missing 2) in the development of a subset of FIHPT cases.

13.4.2. *FHH*

The prevalence of this disorder can reach 1:16,000. Of the roughly 200 mutations in the CASR gene that have been identified, most result in a single missense mutation, creating a receptor protein with relative insensitivity to serum calcium levels.

13.4.3. *NSHPT*

NSHPT is often caused by a homozygous loss of function of the CASR. More than 25 different mutations have been reported in affected patients, and approximately 40% are nonsense or frameshift, leading to truncated CASR.

13.5. Monitoring

Patients with FHH rarely have symptoms of hypercalcemia (constipation, nephrolithiasis, nephrocalcinosis, bone pain, etc.) and hyperparathyroidism. Pancreatitis and chondrocalcinosis are documented complications of FHH, although they are also rare. Since the natural history of FHH is generally benign, patients should not undergo routine subtotal parathyroidectomy or aggressive interventions unless they have a rare localized adenoma or persistent symptomatic hypercalcemia.

14

Hamartomatous Polyposis Syndromes

Hamartomatous polyposis syndromes (HPS) include a small but significant number of hereditary gastrointestinal (GI) cancer syndromes that are characterized by the presence of GI hamartomatous polyps. HPS mainly include PTEN-hamartoma tumor syndromes (PHTS), juvenile polyposis syndrome (JPS) and Peutz–Jeghers syndrome (PJS), although hamartomatous polyps have also been reported in other syndromes (see Figure 4.1). They are transmitted in an autosomal dominant pattern.

14.1. PTEN-hamartoma tumor syndromes

14.1.1. *Introduction*

PHTS include Cowden syndrome (CS), Bannayan–Riley–Ruvalcaba syndrome (BRRS) and PTEN-related Proteus syndrome and Proteus-like syndrome. PTEN-related Proteus syndrome and Proteus-like syndrome are particularly rare overgrowth syndromes and are not yet well understood and will therefore not be discussed here.

14.1.1.1. *Cowden syndrome*

CS is characterized by the presence of multiple hamartomas of the skin and mucous membranes, mucocutaneous lesions, macrocephaly and an increased risk of benign and malignant lesions of the breast, thyroid and endometrium.

14.1.1.2. *Bannayan–Riley–Ruvalcaba syndrome*

BRRS is characterized by macrocephaly, developmental delay, lipomatosis, GI hamartomatous polyps, hemangiomatosis and pigmented macules on the glans penis in men.

14.1.2. *Gene*

PTEN (phosphatase and tensin homolog deleted on chromosome 10) is a tumor suppressor gene that functions primarily as a cellular lipid phosphatase, although in the nucleus it also acts directly as a protein phosphatase and a negative regulator of the mitogen-activated protein kinase (MAPK) pathway.

A number of individuals with CS or CS-like (CSL) characteristics have no detectable germline mutation in PTEN. A number of other possible candidate genes have been identified (SDH, KLLN, EGFR, SEC23B and USF3).

14.1.3. *Tumors*

14.1.3.1. *CS*

It has been estimated that patients with CS have a lifetime risk of cancer of 85.2% for breast cancer, 35.2% for thyroid cancer, 28% for endometrial cancer, 9% for colorectal cancer, 33.6% for kidney cancer and 6% for melanoma.

It has been shown that PTEN mutations and SDH variants are not necessarily mutually exclusive in CS/CSL individuals and that the risk of breast cancer appears to be higher when both are present, as opposed to PTEN mutations alone.

14.1.3.2. *BRRS*

Hamartomatous polyps have been reported in approximately 45% of patients with BRRS, particularly in the ileum and colon. However, these polyps are not thought to increase the risk of GI cancer.

Carriers of PTEN germline mutations (approximately 60%) have a similar risk of malignancy as those with CS.

14.1.4. *Genetics*

The incidence is estimated at 1/200,000 live births, although this is considered an underestimate due to under-diagnosis. It is believed that more than 90% of individuals with germline mutations in PTEN will be symptomatic by age 20 and 100% by age 30.

14.1.5. *Monitoring*

It is important for clinicians to recognize the phenotypic (especially extracolic) features associated with HPS in general and PHTS in particular, as well as the confounding factors that make diagnoses difficult, so that they can offer genetic counseling to their patients when appropriate. Since many pathognomonic features of BRRS and CS are age-dependent, a low threshold for molecular testing in children with macrocephaly and neurodevelopmental disorder or hamartomatous polyps is thought to be particularly important for future medical management and appropriate genetic counseling for the family.

Given the different risks of cancers related to the disease it is advisable to carry out the following examinations:

– breast: a clinical examination of the breasts twice a year from the age of 25 and a mammogram, or even a breast MRI once a year from the age of 30–35;

– endometrium: a transvaginal ultrasound and an annual endometrial biopsy at the age of 30–35 years;

– thyroid cancer (mainly follicular): clinical examinations and ultrasound at diagnosis on an annual basis;

– colon: a colonoscopy from the age of 35 every five years (rhythm to be adjusted according to the results of the first colonoscopy);

– melanoma: an annual dermatological examination from the age of 15;

– kidney cancer: a kidney ultrasound every 1–2 years from the age of 40.

14.2. Juvenile polyposis syndrome

14.2.1. *Introduction*

JPS is characterized by the presence of multiple juvenile hamartomatous polyps in the GI tract, although they are most commonly found in the colon and rectum. Juvenile polyps are lobulated and spherical in shape and are characterized histologically by the proliferation of an edematous lamina propria with inflammatory cells and enlarged cystic glands. Diagnosis is made between 16 and 18 years of age on average, although there is variability in the age of onset and 50% have a family history. Approximately 20% of patients with JPS have manifestations other than hamartomatous polyposis, including congenital anomalies of the heart, skull and sex-urinary systems, cleft lip and palate, clubbing, polydactyly, macrotia, hypertelorism and malrotation of the bowel.

14.2.2. *Gene*

Two genes are currently known to cause JPS: BMPR1A, a type 1 receptor of the transforming growth factor beta super family (TGF-β), located at 10q22.3, and SMAD4, a tumor suppressor gene, located at 18q21.2. Approximately 40–60% of individuals with JPS will carry a germline mutation in the SMAD4 or BMPR1A genes. Large deletions account for 14% of the mutations detected and a further 10% are in the BMPR1A promoter region.

The two proteins encoded by SMAD4 and BMPR1A act in the TGF-β pathway, which is involved in many cellular processes, including growth, differentiation, apoptosis and cell homeostasis.

14.2.3. *Tumors*

The lifetime risk of developing colorectal cancer or cancer of the upper GI tract (mainly gastric) is estimated at 38% and 21%, respectively. The median age of diagnosis is reported to be 42 years. Cancers of the colon and stomach are the most common diseases seen in JPS, although a small number of individuals with JPS have cancers of the pancreas, small intestine, duodenum and jejunum.

14.2.4. *Genetics*

The estimated incidence is one per 100,000 live births. Juvenile polyposis of infancy occurs very early in life (usually at the age of 2) and is the rarest form of JPS. Patients in this group generally have a poor prognosis. They usually have recurrent GI bleeding, diarrhea, hypoproteinemia and malnutrition, as well as larger recurrent polyps that cause rectal prolapse and intestinal invagination. In addition, many suffer from congenital anomalies, including macrocephaly and generalized hypotonia. This severe phenotype is thought to be the result of a contiguous deletion of the BMPR1A and PTEN genes.

Juvenile polyposis coli and generalized JPS are associated with varied expression and penetrance, with polyps usually found in the colon. Symptoms of these forms tend to appear in the second decade of life and the number of polyps may vary throughout the lifetime.

A genotype–phenotype correlation has been reported in which mutations in the SMAD4 gene are associated with a higher risk of large gastric polyps and a higher risk of upper GI malignancy than those in the BMPR1A gene (when JPS is the result of a SMAD4 germline mutation, individuals are at a higher risk of large gastric polyps and malignancy in the upper GI tract than when due to a BMPR1A mutation).

14.2.5. *Monitoring*

The objective of monitoring is to reduce polyposis-related morbidity:

– colon: a colonoscopy from the age of 15 every two years (this is changed to annually as soon as the first polyp is detected). A colectomy should be considered if the number of polyps is too high;

– cancers of the upper GI tract: a GI endoscopy from the age of 15 every two years (this is changed to annually as soon as the first polyp is detected).

14.3. Peutz–Jeghers syndrome

14.3.1. *Introduction*

PJS is characterized by the presence of hamartomatous polyps of the Peutz–Jeghers type in the GI tract and mucocutaneous pigmentation. Peutz–Jeghers polyps have a distinct slingshot-like structure, an epithelium and smooth muscle proliferating into the lamina propria.

Histologically, Peutz–Jeghers polyps have elongated convolutional glands and a tree-branching pattern of smooth muscle growth. The number of polyps can vary from one to several hundred and they appear most often in the small intestine, but also frequently in the colon and stomach.

Mucocutaneous pigmentation is present in approximately 95% of individuals with PJS and is found on the vermilion edge of the lips, the oral mucosa and the perianal region.

14.3.2. *Gene*

PJS is caused by the presence of germline mutations in the STK11 tumor suppressor gene (LKB1) located at 19p13.3. It is 23 kb in size, consists of ten exons (nine of which are coding) and encodes a 433 amino acid STK (serine threonine kinase) protein.

The STK11/LKB1 gene regulates cell polarity and acts as a tumor suppressor. LKB1 is a primary kinase upstream of AMPK (adenine monophosphate-activated protein kinase), a necessary component of cellular metabolism and crucial for the maintenance of energy homeostasis.

Activation of AMPK by LKB1 inhibits growth and proliferation when energy and nutrient levels are scarce. Activation of AMPK-related kinases by LKB1 plays a critical role in maintaining cell polarity, thereby inhibiting inappropriate tumor cell expansion.

14.3.3. *Tumors*

The cumulative lifetime risk for any cancer in PJS has been estimated to be 89%. The most common cancers identified in patients with PJS are those located in the GI tract, including the esophagus, stomach, small intestine, colon and pancreas. Breast cancer in women is also frequently reported, although some argue that the degree of risk may not be as high as commonly cited.

Also associated with PJS are cancers of the reproductive organs. Women are at increased risk of developing sex cord tumors with annular tubules of the ovary and malignant adenoma of the cervix. Men have an increased risk of developing sex cord and Sertoli cell type testicular tumors, often resulting in sexual precocity and gynecomastia.

DEFINITION.– Gynecomastia *is an increase in the amount of breast gland tissue in boys or men caused by an imbalance of the hormones estrogen and testosterone. Gynecomastia can affect one or both breasts, sometimes unevenly.*

14.3.4. *Genetics*

The incidence of PJS is approximately 1/8,300 to 1/230,000 live births, although a more recent report estimates the lower limit at 1/50,000.

The mutation detection rate in individuals meeting the diagnostic criteria for PJS is 94% when using sequencing and MLPA (multiplex ligation-dependent probe amplification). Approximately 38–50% of individuals with a constitutional STK11 mutation do not have a family history of PJS.

The majority of mutations associated with the disease are truncated or missense mutations that eliminate the protein's kinase function. Importantly, up to 30% of mutations can be large deletions that are often not detected by sequencing alone.

There are conflicting reports regarding genotype–phenotype correlations. Parents of apparently *de novo* cases need to be carefully assessed for the characteristics of PJS.

14.3.5. *Monitoring*

Although there is little evidence documenting the effectiveness of monitoring of individuals with PJS, recommendations have been developed based on expert opinion:

– colon: a colonoscopy from the age of 25 every two to three years;

– cancers of the upper GI tract/small intestine: a GI endoscopy from the age of ten, every two to three years, or video capsule endoscopy (VCE), barium follow through (BaFT) or magnetic resonance endoscopy (MRE); an annual hemoglobin test in childhood;

– pancreatic cancer: an endoscopic ultrasound and a trans-abdominal ultrasound every one to two years starting at age 30;

– breast cancer: a mammogram every one to two years and an annual palpation of the breasts from the age of 25;

– gynecological cancer/tumors: an annual transvaginal ultrasound and endometrial biopsy from the age of 20. A cervico uterine smear and annual pelvic examination from the age of 18–20 years;

– testicular cancer: a physical examination and an ultrasound if clinically indicated at an annual rate starting at age ten.

15

Fanconi Syndrome

15.1. Introduction

Fanconi anemia (FA) is characterized by birth defects, progressive bone marrow failure and an increased risk of cancer in early adulthood.

Symptoms that may lead physicians to suspect FA include a variety of congenital abnormalities, including microcephaly, microphthalmia, abnormal thumbs or radial ray abnormalities and slow growth rate.

Hematological signs may include early aplastic anemia, myelodysplastic syndrome (MDS), acute myeloid leukemia (AML) at an atypical young age and one or more unexplained cytopenias of all cell lines, including thrombocytopenia, neutropenia and anemia.

DEFINITION.– Neutropenia *is a condition in which there is a lower than normal number of neutrophils (a type of white blood cell) in the blood.*

DEFINITION.– Thrombocytopenia *is a condition in which the number of platelets in the blood is lower than normal. This can lead to easy bruising and excessive bleeding from wounds or bleeding into mucous membranes and other tissues.*

In addition, attention should be paid to the presentation of solid tumors at a particularly young age, especially squamous cell carcinomas of the head, neck, esophagus and gynecological organs. Family predisposition to cancer or a history of chemotherapeutic hypersensitivity may also raise suspicion of FA.

15.2. Gene

The speed of identification of FA genes has increased rapidly. With the most recent additions, there are now 21 confirmed FA genes: FANCA, FANCB, FANCC, BRCA2/FANCD1, FANCD2, FANCE, FANCF, FANCG, FANCI, BRIP1/FANCJ, FANCL, FANCM, PALB2/FANCN, RAD51C/FANCO, SLX4/FANCP, ERCC4/FANCQ and, more recently, RAD51/FANCR, BRCA1/FANCS, UBE2T/FANCT, XRCC2/FANCU and MAD2L2/REV7/FANCV.

All FA genes are involved in the FA-BRCA pathway. One of the main functions of the FA-BRCA pathway is to orchestrate the repair of interstrand cross-links (ICL) in DNA. Examples of ICL-inducing agents include diepoxybutane (DEB) and mitomycin C (MMC).

ICLs are a direct physical blockage of DNA replication and RNA transcription and lead to cellular cytotoxicity and structural aberrations of chromosomes if not properly repaired. Cells from FA patients have a characteristic hypersensitivity to ICL, and this phenotype is the basis for the clinical diagnostic test for FA. In particular, cells from FA patients show an increased formation of radial chromosomes after the induction of ICL as a consequence of molecular impediment to ICL repair.

15.3. Tumors

It has been reported that the overall risks of leukemia and solid tumors in FA cohorts are approximately 30–50 times greater; the highest risks include AML, head and neck squamous cell carcinoma (HNSCC) and squamous cell carcinoma of the vulva.

15.4. Genetics

FA is primarily an autosomal recessive disorder with at least 21 associated DNA repair genes. Pathogenic variants of an X-linked recessive gene, FANCB, and an autosomal dominant gene, FANCR/RAD51, have been reported.

With an estimated incidence of 1/360,000 live births and a carrier frequency of approximately 1/181, FA is relatively rare and can be difficult to diagnose because patients present with a wide variety of symptoms.

15.5. Monitoring

A complete blood count (CBC) and bone marrow biopsy are recommended at the time of diagnosis. The bone marrow assessment should then be repeated annually. The CBC should be monitored more frequently to allow for proactive monitoring of progressive cytopenias and MDS. Starting from diagnosis time, patients with FA should have a monthly oral self-examination (or with parental assistance) and undergo a biennial dental examination (general inspection without radiography unless specifically indicated) and an annual HNSCC evaluation by an otolaryngologist in early adolescence. An annual gynecological examination is recommended starting in adolescence and HPV vaccination should be given for both boys and girls. Clinical management of patients with FA does not include standard myeloablative dosing, but rather a reduced-intensity conditioning (RIC), as these low-dose regimens are designed to be myeloablative for FA; alternatively, androgen therapy may be tried for patients with FA with medullary insufficiency, as well as specific treatment of cancer by avoiding DNA-damaging agents.

Parents of children with the more common subtypes of FA, FANCA, FANCC and FANCG do not appear to have an increased risk of cancer. However, heterozygous mutations in several of the rarer subtypes of FA genes (FANCD1/BRCA2, FANCJ/BRIP1, FANCN/PALB2, FANCO/RAD51C, FANCS/ BRCA1 and FANCU/XRCC2) are associated with moderate risks of cancer in adults, particularly for breast and ovarian cancer. Thus, parents of children with these subtypes should benefit from appropriate strategies for screening and prevention of the cancers in question.

16

Hereditary Diffuse Gastric Cancer

16.1. Introduction

Hereditary diffuse gastric cancer (HDGC) is an autosomal dominant disease described by Guilford in 1998. HDGC is due to mutations in the E-cadherin gene.

The E-cadherin (CDH1) gene has been identified in about 40% of families with an HDGC-compatible pedigree and with a penetrance of about 80%, which is compatible with an autosomal dominant mode of transmission. HDGC patients may also be predisposed to lobular breast cancer.

16.2. Gene

The CDH1 gene is located on chromosome 16q22.1. It consists of 16 exons transcribed into a 4.5 kb mRNA and codes for E-cadherin. E-cadherin is a calcium-dependent cell–cell adhesion molecule that plays a crucial role in establishing epithelial architecture and maintaining cell polarity and differentiation. In addition to its role in cell–cell adhesion, E-cadherin is involved in a number of signaling pathways in carcinogenesis. Since the negative regulation of E-cadherin in epithelial cells results in reduced cell polarity and increased migratory and invasive growth properties, the loss of E-cadherin stimulates the active signals that initiate epithelial mesenchymal transition (EMT).

16.3. Tumors

Hereditary gastric cancer accounts for approximately 1–3% of all cases of gastric adenocarcinoma. HDGC is characterized by signet ring cell carcinomas and is considered to be a type of cancer with a poor prognosis.

The presence of a CDH1 mutation will result in an 80% cumulative risk of gastric cancer for men and women at age 80 and a 60% cumulative risk of lobular breast cancer for women at age 80. There is no significantly increased risk for other types of cancer, but there is growing evidence of an increased risk of colon cancer.

16.4. Genetics

The germline mutations in the CDH1 gene, which encodes E-cadherin, were the first HDGC mutations discovered. Loss of E-cadherin expression has been linked to tumor progression, invasion and metastasis. The mechanisms of genetic inactivation of E-cadherin in HDGC are diverse, including rearrangements and mutations of frameshift, splice site, missense and nonsense. Promoter hypermethylation is the most common cause of a "second hit" that inactivates the wild-type allele and initiates tumorigenesis.

Other potential candidate HDGC susceptibility genes have been suggested and include CTNNA1, INSR, FBXO24, MAP3K6, CD44, DOT1L, PALB2, BRCA1, RAD51C and MET.

16.5. Monitoring

Patients with the CDH1 mutation may benefit from endoscopic monitoring to determine the timing of surgery. The NCCN guidelines recommend prophylactic gastrectomy for carriers of CDH1 pathogenic mutations. However, individuals who refuse such treatment may consider gastroscopic monitoring with multiple biopsies every 6–12 months after genetic counseling.

It has been suggested that it is preferable to adjust the start time for monitoring among carriers of the CDH1 mutation (to age 20) and non-carrier family members who are at risk (to age 40).

With respect to the age of prophylactic gastrectomy, the NCCN estimates that the earliest age for prophylactic gastrectomy in general is 18 years, while others suggest that the earliest optimal age is 20 years.

A total gastrectomy was performed on a 16-year-old asymptomatic CDH1 mutation carrier. Two normal gastroscopy results with biopsies prior to gastrectomy were obtained. However, several foci of early-stage carcinoma were found in his gastrectomy sample. The family history showed that the patient's mother and aunt died at 39 and 21 years of age, respectively, both of stomach cancer. This illustrates the limitations of gastroscopic monitoring and also the need to adjust the age of prophylactic gastric bypass surgery based on family history.

DEFINITION.– Gastrectomy *is an operation to remove all or part of the stomach.*

Annual monitoring endoscopy starting 5–10 years before the earliest age of diagnosis of cancer in the family should be offered in a specialized center with endoscopists and pathologists experienced in this type of case.

In view of the high risk of lobular breast cancer, it has been recommended that women aged 35 years and older be monitored for breast cancer with annual mammography, breast MRI and clinical breast examination every six months. Based on emerging evidence of colon cancer in this population (HDGC criteria), colonoscopy has been recommended from age 40 onwards.

17

Von Hippel–Lindau Disease

17.1. Introduction

Von Hippel–Lindau (VHL) syndrome is an autosomal dominant familial neoplastic multiorgan syndrome caused by genetic aberrations in the VHL tumor suppressor gene.

Germline mutations in the VHL gene predispose affected individuals to the development of benign and malignant tumors in several systems, including the central nervous system (CNS) and visceral organs such as the kidneys, pancreas, adrenal glands and reproductive organs.

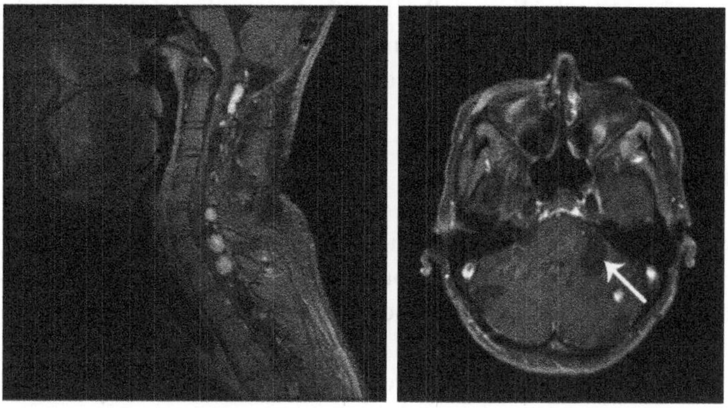

a) b)

Figure 17.1. *VHL, hemangioblastoma. For a color version of this figure, see www.iste.co.uk/boukhatem/oncogenetics.zip*

COMMENT ON FIGURE 17.1.– *(a) Sagittal view of the neck of an individual showing several light-colored lesions along the spinal cord. Hemangioblastomas are the most common manifestation of the disease in patients with VHL syndrome. Several hemangioblastomas of the spinal cord are shown; (b) axial view of an individual's head showing a light-colored lesion in the cerebellum with a large dark area, which is a cystic component. A cerebellar lesion (red arrow) is shown with a dominant cystic component (white arrow).*

17.2. Gene

The VHL gene is located on the short arm of chromosome 3 (3p25-26). It codes for pVHL, a tumor suppressor protein involved in cellular signaling pathways. There are two isoforms of pVHL: pVHL30 and pVHL19. Both isoforms are important for normal function of VHL.

pVHL plays an important role in the hydroxylation of HIF-α (hypoxia-inducible factor 1 alpha) under normoxic conditions. In VHL, the VHL gene becomes non-functional. The absence of the functional VHL gene results in hyperaccumulation of HIF-α, which can lead to excessive activation of many hypoxia-inducible genes, including vascular endothelial growth factor (VEGF), platelet-derived growth factor (PDGF), transforming growth factor alpha (TGFα), glucose transporter 1 (GLUT1) and phosphofructokinase 1 (PFK-1).

Factors induced in the hypoxia/VHL pathway are thought to play a key role in the pathogenesis of VHL-related tumors. Excessive uncontrolled angiogenesis contributes to the hypervascular nature of tumors that develop in this state.

17.3. Tumors

Patients can develop multiple benign and malignant tumors involving various organs, including retinal hemangioblastomas (HBs), CNS, endolymphatic sac tumors, pancreatic neuroendocrine tumors, pancreatic cystadenomas, pancreatic cysts, clear cell renal cell carcinomas (RCCs), renal cysts, pheochromocytomas (PCCs), paragangliomas, and epididymal and broad ligament cystadenomas.

DEFINITION.– *The* cystadenoma *is a rare benign cystic epithelial neoplasm that frequently contains epithelium-lined papillary projections in the cystic spaces.*

DEFINITION.– *The* epididymis *is a tightly coiled tube about 600 cm long where sperm matures as it passes through.*

CNS hemangioblastomas are the most common tumors of VHL syndrome and affect 60–80% of all patients. The average age of presentation is 33 years. These tumors are benign, but are a major cause of morbidity and mortality due to the mass effect on structures adjacent to the CNS.

Retinal hemangioblastoma is common in patients with VHL. They are seen in 60% of patients.

Endolymphatic sac tumors (ELST) develop from the endolymphatic epithelium in the vestibular aqueduct. These tumors are present in 6–15% of patients with VHL. However, they are rare in the general population. They usually appear around the age of 31 years. They are benign tumors that do not metastasize, but may be locally aggressive.

Renal manifestations of VHL include benign renal cysts and clear cell carcinoma. Multiple bilateral renal cysts are found at screening in 50–70% of patients with VHL. RCC can affect up to 30% of patients with VHL. Bilateral RCC and renal cysts develop in the third or fourth decade of life in these patients. Up to 70% of patients with VHL develop RCC by the age of 60.

PCCs occur in up to 20% of VHL patients. They can be bilateral and sometimes multifocal. PCCs are usually present in the second decade of life in patients with VHL and rarely develop into malignancies.

Approximately 35–70% of patients with VHL have pancreatic lesions. Up to 72% of VHL patients have pancreatic cysts at autopsy. Serous cystadenomas and neuroendocrine tumors are other manifestations of pancreatic lesions in VHL syndrome. Neuroendocrine tumors may become malignant and metastatic in 8% of patients.

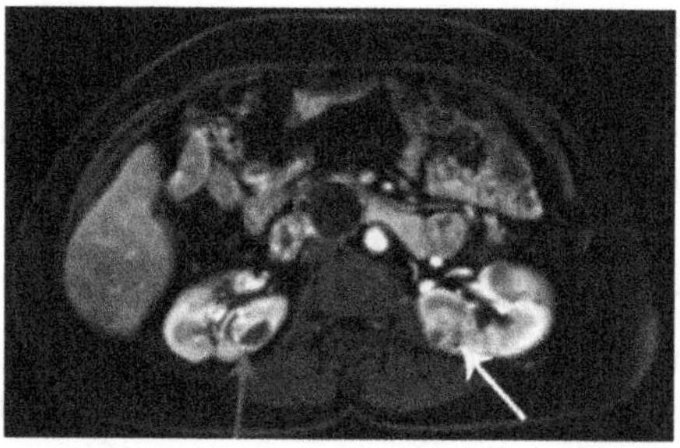

Figure 17.2. *VHL, renal tumors, bilateral. For a color version of this figure, see www.iste.co.uk/boukhatem/oncogenetics.zip*

COMMENT ON FIGURE 17.2.– *Axial view of the mid-section of an individual showing tumors in both kidneys. The left kidney has a tumor with a dark cystic component and the right kidney has a predominantly solid tumor. RCC associated with VHL are typically multifocal and bilateral and present as a combined cystic and solid mass. The red arrow (left) indicates a lesion with a solid and cystic component and the white arrow (right) indicates a predominantly solid lesion.*

17.4. Genetics

Missense mutations (27–52%) are the most common type of germline mutation in VHL. However, a broad spectrum of germline mutations has been described, including frameshift mutations, nonsense mutations, large deletions or microdeletions, gene rearrangements, deletions or insertions in the frame and splice site mutations.

Specific genotype–phenotype correlations in the affected families have led to the classification of HSV subtypes into types 1 and 2, mainly on the basis of the presence of PCC. Type 1 diseases have a very low risk of PCCs while type 2 diseases have an increased risk of PCCs. Type 2 VHLs are also classified as type 2a (low risk of RCC), type 2b (high risk of RCC) and type 2c with PCCs only.

Approximately 80% of patients diagnosed with VHL have an affected relative. Approximately 20% of individuals do not have a positive family history and have a *de novo* pathogenic variant.

17.5. Monitoring

The management of VHL-associated tumors requires a multidisciplinary approach. Various follow-up guidelines have been put in place to help monitor the progression of the various manifestations of VHL. In particular, the prevention of kidney cancer by appropriate monitoring of renal cysts whose malignant transformation is slow proved to be effective.

Monitoring can begin as early as one year of age, as described below.

1) 1–4 years: ohthalmological follow-up at an annual rate (eye or retinal examination with indirect ophthalmoscopy) and a thorough clinical examination to look for signs of neurological disorders (nystagmus, white pupil) and anomalies in blood pressure, hearing or vision.

DEFINITION.– Nystagmus *is a generally rapid involuntary movement of the eyeballs (such as from side to side) normally occurring with dizziness during and after body rotation or abnormally following head trauma or as a symptom of disease.*

2) 5–15 years:

– annual examinations:

- physical examination and neurological evaluation for blood pressure (lying and standing), hearing problems, neurological disturbance, nystagmus, strabismus, white pupils and other signs,

- ocular or retinal examination with indirect ophthalmoscopy,

- abdominal ultrasound every year from the age of eight years if required,

- testing for plasma metanephrines or 24 h urinary metanephrines;

– every 2–3 years:

- full hearing assessment,

- if ear infections are reoccurring, magnetic resonance imaging (MRI) with internal ear canal contrast for possible ELST.

3) 16 years old and older:

– annual examinations:

- thorough physical examination,

- ocular or retinal examination with indirect ophthalmoscopy,

- ultrasound and MRI of the abdomen with and without contrast to assess the kidneys, pancreas and adrenal glands,

- testing for plasma metanephrines or 24 h urinary metanephrines;

– every two years:

- MRI with cervical, thoracic and lumbar spine contrast to eliminate both ELST and hemangioblastoma,

- hearing assessment.

18

Xeroderma Pigmentosum

18.1. Introduction

Xeroderma pigmentosum (XP) is a photosensitive genetic disorder in which patients have a high sensitivity to skin cancer at sun-exposed body sites.

Approximately 60% of those affected have an exaggerated and prolonged response to sunburn. In a minority of cases, there are neurological abnormalities of varying severity. XP is a genetic disease in which genetic abnormalities occur in the DNA repair process. XP patients easily develop several skin cancers if they are not completely protected from UV radiation.

XP is classified into the following types: XP skin disease in which patients develop only skin symptoms; XP neurological disease in which patients develop skin symptoms with neurological symptoms; and XP/Cockayne syndrome in which patients develop skin symptoms along with those of CS (very rare).

DEFINITION.– Cockayne syndrome (CS) *is a genetic condition characterized by short stature, premature aging, sensitivity to light, and possibly deafness and intellectual disability.*

18.2. Gene

XP occurs because the repair system (nucleotide excision repair (NER) and translesion synthesis repair) of UV-induced DNA damage (cyclo-butane-type pyrimidine dimer, 6-4 photoproduct) does not work properly due to a genetic abnormality. The genes responsible are XPA, XPB (ERCC3), XPC, XPD (ERCC2), XPE (DDB2), XPF (ERCC4), XPG (ERCC5) and XPV (POLH). All are

NER-related factors except for the XPV protein, which performs the translesion DNA polymerase function in the translesion synthetic repair system.

The products of seven of these genes (XP-A to G) are involved in the repair of ultraviolet induced photoproducts in DNA by the NER process.

The proteins XPC and XPE are needed to recognize photoproducts in DNA. XPB and XPD are part of a TFIIH protein complex, which opens up the structure of DNA around the site of the photoproduct. The XPA protein verifies that the proteins are in the correct position, and then the XPG and XPF nuclease cut the DNA on either side of the damage, so that the damaged section can be removed and replaced with intact DNA.

18.3. Tumors

In the absence of strict sun protection, areas of hyper- and hypopigmentation will result, followed by accelerated photoaging, warty lesions, malignant tumors of melanocytes and keratinocytes *in situ* and possibly several basal cell carcinomas and invasive squamous cell carcinomas and melanomas.

It has been estimated that XP patients under 20 years of age have a 10,000 times higher risk of non-melanoma skin cancer and a 2,000 times higher risk of melanoma.

18.4. Genetics

XP is an inherited photosensitive disease with an autosomal recessive mode of transmission. Estimates suggest an incidence in the United States of 1:250,000 and in Japan of 1:20,000. In Western Europe, estimates are about 2.3 per million live births. XP is an autosomal recessive disorder with 100% penetrance and can result from mutations in one of eight genes.

18.5. Monitoring

Although no cure is available for XP, skin problems can be considerably improved with appropriate protection. However, some of the effects of sun exposure prior to diagnosis may manifest themselves years later despite adequate sun protection after diagnosis. Since skin changes are all caused by ultraviolet radiation, complete protection from ultraviolet exposure can prevent further skin changes.

As with all genetic disorders, genetic counseling is appropriate for families to discuss the etiology, the likelihood of occurrence in future pregnancies and the increased likelihood of occurrence in communities where consanguineous marriages are common.

DEFINITION.– Consanguinity *is a genetic relationship between individuals descended from at least one common ancestor.*

Regular visits should be made to the dermatologist so that any precancerous lesions can be removed as soon as possible. Frequent eye examinations by an ophthalmologist are recommended. Strict sun protection can lead to vitamin D deficiency; therefore, vitamin D supplements should be prescribed.

19

Hereditary Papillary Renal Carcinoma

19.1. Introduction

Hereditary papillary renal carcinoma (HPRC) is subdivided into two types. In type 1, papillary type 1 tumors develop weakly. In contrast to this type of relatively slow-growing tumor, in type 2 the tumors associated with hereditary leiomyomatosis and renal cell cancer (HLRCC) are among the most aggressive.

HPRC type 1 is caused by an activating mutation of the proto-oncogene MET located on chromosome 7q31.2. HLRCC is caused by a mutation in the fumarate hydratase (FH) gene located at 1q42.3-q43.

19.2. Gene

19.2.1. *MET*

MET codes for a transmembrane protein, which is the receptor for hepatocyte growth factor tyrosine kinase, also known as dispersion factor. The proto-oncogenic product c-Met is a receptor-like tyrosine kinase consisting of two disulfide bonded subunits, one of 50 kD (alpha) and other of 145 kD (beta). In the mature c-Met product, the alpha subunit is extracellular and the beta subunit has extracellular, transmembrane and tyrosine kinase domains and tyrosine phosphorylation sites.

19.2.2. *FH*

The protein encoded by the FH gene is an enzyme component of the tricarboxylic acid cycle (TCA), or Krebs cycle, and is the catalyst for the formation of L-malate from fumarate. It exists in both a cytosolic and an N-terminal extended form, differing only in the site of translation initiation used. The N-terminal extended form is addressed to the mitochondrion, where suppression of extension generates the same form as in the cytoplasm. It is similar to some thermostable class II fumarases and functions as a homotetramer.

19.3. Tumors

19.3.1. *HPRC*

HPRC induce type 1 papillary tumors, with as many as 3,400 tumors per kidney, although most are microscopic. Most tumors are too small to be seen without a microscope, but macroscopic tumors can also appear and be visible by imaging. Removal of a tumor is recommended at a diameter of 3 cm to avoid metastatic disease which, although rare, can occur. Type 1 papillary renal tumors tend to grow slowly and therefore do not appear until 50–70 years of age during life and frequently only at autopsy.

No other tumors or manifestations are known in HPRC, making it unique among hereditary kidney cancers.

19.3.2. *HLRCC*

HLRCC induce type 2 papillary renal tumors. Approximately 15–30% of patients with an FH mutation develop kidney cancer. The average age of reporting is 36–39 years. Tumor cells have a large nucleus with a prominent organiophilic or eosinophilic nucleolus surrounded by a clear halo. These tumors grow aggressively unlike most other kidney cancers.

HLRCC was first discovered in women with what appeared to be a predisposition to uterine leiomyomas. Uterine fibroids develop at 20–35 years of age and patients often require a hysterectomy because of presentation of aggressive growth with symptoms of menorrhagia and pelvic pain. Patients also develop cutaneous leiomyomas that can be painful at pressure or low temperature and located on the trunk and limbs. These lesions, whether on the skin or in the uterus, generally remain benign, but malignant changes have been reported. Adrenal cortical hyperplasia has been reported in some cases of HLRCC.

DEFINITION.– Menorrhagia *is abnormally heavy menstrual bleeding.*

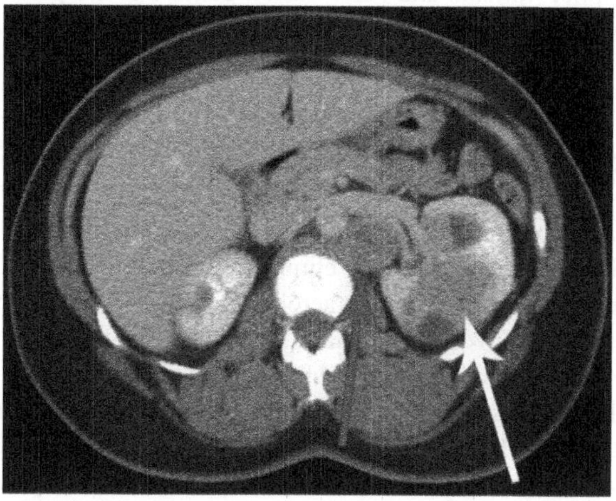

Figure 19.1. *HLRCC, renal tumor. For a color version of this figure, see www.iste.co.uk/boukhatem/oncogenetics.zip*

COMMENT ON FIGURE 19.1.– *Axial view of the mid-section of an individual showing tumors in both kidneys. The left kidney has a small tumor and the right kidney has a larger tumor. A retroperitoneal lymph node is shown next to the larger tumor. Renal tumors associated with HLRCC are usually unilateral and solitary; in a few individuals, they are multifocal. The red arrow (left) indicates a retroperitoneal lymph node. The white arrow (right) indicates a left kidney mass.*

19.4. Genetics

19.4.1. *HPRC type 1*

HPRC type 1 is an autosomal dominant disease with high penetrance. It is a rare disease with an estimated incidence of one in 10 million. Only 30 known families have been described. Two-thirds of affected patients develop papillary kidney cancer by the age of 60 and 90% by the age of 80, indicating high penetrance.

Mutations in the tyrosine kinase part of the receptor cause activation leading to cell proliferation, prolonged cell survival, increased cell motility and angiogenesis. In HPRC, trisomy 7 with duplication of the mutant MET allele can cause disease.

Mutations, splice variants and MET fusion genes that are predicted to activate the MET pathway can be observed in 15% of cases of sporadic papillary type 1 RCC.

19.4.2. *HLRCC*

HLRCC is an autosomal dominant disease. Mutations in FH cause an interruption of the normal Krebs cycle, effectively eliminating oxidative phosphorylation in the cells and causing a metabolic switch to aerobic glycolysis (Warburg physiology). As fumarate is no longer converted to malate, fumarate accumulates in the cell, acting as a competitive inhibitor of HIF-prolyl hydroxylase, thus preventing degradation of HIF by VHL. The increase in intracellular glucose levels, caused by the metabolism of glucose outside the Krebs cycle, produces NADPH-mediated reactive oxygen species that also further stabilize HIF. This results in the creation of a pseudo-hypoxic state similar to VHL, which promotes cell growth.

19.5. Monitoring

19.5.1. *HPRC*

HPRC tumors are slow growing and usually painless. Therefore, they do not require frequent monitoring. Imaging follow-up every 2–4 years with MRI is recommended in affected family members, but the frequency can be adjusted to the proliferative profile if it is very slow.

19.5.2. *HLRCC*

Due to their aggressive behavior, HLRCC tumors are not monitored. They are treated as soon as they can be verified. An annual MRI examination for patients with no signs of kidney failure but with a positive genetic screening can detect tumors at an early stage while they are still curable. Once a tumor is identified for surgery, either by radical nephrectomy or partial nephrectomy, wide surgical margins are recommended for any solid mass of HLRCC. The 3 cm rule does not apply to HLRCC.

DEFINITION.– Nephrectomy *is surgery to remove a kidney or part of a kidney. In a partial nephrectomy, a part of a kidney or a tumor is removed, but not a whole kidney. In a simple nephrectomy, one kidney is removed. In a radical nephrectomy, a whole kidney, the nearby adrenal gland and surrounding lymph nodes and other tissue are removed. In a bilateral nephrectomy, both kidneys are removed.*

Other benign lesions (uterine and cutaneous leiomyomas; hyperplasia of the adrenal cortex) should be monitored, as malignant changes cannot be ruled out.

20

Retinoblastoma

20.1. Introduction

Retinoblastoma (RB) is the most common intraocular malignancy in children. Almost two thirds of cases are diagnosed before the age of two years and 95% diagnosed before the age of five years.

RB generally occurs in two forms: hereditary and non-hereditary (sporadic). In hereditary cases, a germline mutation in the RB1 gene predisposes to the development of RB.

20.2. Gene

The RB1 gene codes for the pRB protein. pRB is a nuclear phosphoprotein belonging to the pocket protein family. pRB is a key negatively regulated transcription factor that regulates the cell cycle transition from G1 to S by blocking the interactions of transcription factors E2F and DP (dimerization partner) with DNA. In response to mitogen-stimulated cyclin-dependent kinase signaling, normal pRB is hyperphosphorylated and dissociates from E2F, allowing these factors to activate transcription. pRB also has an increasing spectrum of roles in differentiation, chromatin remodeling, genome stability and apoptosis.

20.3. Tumors

RB is a small-blue-round-cell tumor. It therefore has histological similarity to other tumors of the nervous system in children, including neuroblastoma and medulloblastoma. The cells are mainly composed of large basophilic nuclei and a small cytoplasm. The tumor is very proliferative and has abundant mitosis and necrosis. The cells may take on a polygonal shape and mimic cobblestones when clustered together.

Children with hereditary RB are also at risk of developing a primary intracranial primitive neuroectodermal tumor (PNET), in addition to unilateral, bilateral RB or trilateral RB. These are most often pinealoblastomas, but tumors of the suprasellar or parasellar regions may also occur.

DEFINITION.– Pinealoblastoma *is a type of fast-growing brain tumor that occurs in or around the pineal gland, a tiny organ near the center of the brain. The pineal gland releases melatonin, a hormone that controls sleep.*

The risk of a second malignancy is about 20% in patients with hereditary RB who have not received radiation therapy and significantly higher (40–50%) in those who have been irradiated. The median age of the second primary tumor is between 15 and 17 years.

Melanomas have been reported both within and outside the area of radiation therapy, as well as in irradiated and non-irradiated patients. The median age has been reported at 27 years (range 9.2–37 years).

20.4. Genetics

This is a rare pediatric cancer with an age-adjusted incidence rate of approximately 3–5 per million children in the United States and Europe, although considerable geographic variation has been reported.

Approximately 40% of RBs are hereditary, of which about 80% are derived from *de novo* germline mutations in the absence of a known family history. The majority of hereditary cases have bilateral or multifocal ocular involvement, but about 10–15% of children with unilocal and unifocal RB are also hereditary.

Hereditary RB is inherited in an autosomal dominant mode, with *de novo* mutations in most cases. The majority of germline mutations lead to 90–95% penetrance and carriers generally develop bilateral or multifocal tumors.

Nonsense and frameshift mutations in exons 2–25 almost always lead to a very penetrating bilateral RB, and are the most common type of mutation among family cases. Mutations with low penetrance and variable expressivity have also been described. These include missense mutations, especially those in the less well-preserved residues and in the promoter regions, as well as some splice site mutations.

A small subgroup of individuals with RB has a complete deletion of the gene due to germline deletions of 13q. Although the data are limited, the phenotype RB appears to be the same, and pinealoblastoma has also been reported in this context.

Individuals with these cytogenetic deletions may have dysmorphic facial features (usually anteverted ears, broad forehead, long philtrum) as well as varying levels of neurological impairment.

20.5. Monitoring

Given the high risk of tumor development in carriers of pathogenic RB1 mutations and the positive impact that early detection can have for better visual outcomes, early and intensive intraocular screening is recommended.

20.5.1. *Monitoring for intraocular RB*

This monitoring should begin at birth with an unsedated examination every two weeks until eight weeks of age. After that and up to the age of one year, a monthly examination under anesthesia should be performed, then an examination every two months from 12 to 24 months, an examination every three months from 24 to 36 months, an examination every four months from 36 to 48 months, an examination every six months from 48 to 60 months and an examination every six months from five to seven.

20.5.2. *Monitoring for trilateral RB*

Cerebral magnetic resonance imaging (MRI) at the time of RB diagnosis should be performed; some centers recommend a cerebral MRI every six months for up to five years.

20.5.3. *Monitoring of second primary tumors*

Education about the risk of second primary tumors and special attention to any new signs/symptoms is recommended.

Skin examination by the pediatrician during consultations, to be continued every year by the primary care physician or dermatologist for melanoma screening from the age of 18 years, is recommended.

Genetic counseling plays a critical role in the care of patients with RB. Genetic testing provides families with information about the risk of recurrence and helps guide appropriate recommendations for screening patients and their siblings.

21

Carney Complex

21.1. Introduction

Carney complex (CNC) is a multiple neoplastic syndrome with endocrine and non-endocrine manifestations. Diagnostic criteria include myxoma, lentigines, and primary pigmented nodular adrenal cortical disease, among other signs and symptoms.

DEFINITION.– Myxoma *is a benign tumor of connective tissue containing mucous or gelatinous material. It is most commonly found in the heart, but can also occur in other places. Most myxomas develop in the atria.*

Inactivating mutations in the PRKAR1A gene have been identified as the main cause of the disease, although since 2015 other genes related to the disease have been identified, including activating mutations in PRKACA and PRKACB.

The main endocrine manifestation of CNC is primary pigmented nodular adrenal disease (PPNAD). The latter is a cause of ACTH-independent Cushing's syndrome.

21.2. Gene

The PRKAR1A gene codes for the I-α (RIα) regulatory subunit of cAMP-dependent protein kinase A (PKA) and functions as a tumor suppressor gene. The PKA enzyme complex is the most important intracellular cAMP receptor in eukaryotic cells. The protein kinase modulates the activity of several proteins, inducing phosphorylation of the hydroxyl group in the serine and/or threonine groups of different proteins; it is therefore a serine/threonine-specific protein kinase.

Constitutional Oncogenetics,
Noureddine BOUKHATEM. © ISTE Ltd 2021.

In its inactive state, PKA is a tetrameric complex composed of two regulating subunits (R), type I-α (RI-α) and type II-β (RII-β), and two catalytic subunits (C), type I-α (CI-α) and type II-β (CII-β).

The binding of cAMP to the two sites of a subunit (R) leads to the release of the associated subunit (C), revealing its catalytic site and activating its kinase action. The best known function attributed to subunits (R) is the inhibition of the kinase activity of subunits (C). The release of the catalytic subunits (C) from the PKA complex is followed by their translocation to the cell nucleus, with phosphorylation of CREB proteins in serine-threonine phosphorylation substrates in response to increased levels of cAMP. Inactivating mutations in the PRKAR1A gene in the CNC result in amplification of the cAMP signal.

PKA is extensively involved in various cellular processes, including transcription, metabolism, cell cycle progression and apoptosis.

Other genes also involved in CNC are genes coding for the alpha catalytic subunit of protein kinase A complex (PRKACA) and for the beta catalytic subunit of protein kinase A complex (PRKACB).

21.3. Tumors

PPNAD causing Cushing's syndrome of adrenal origin is the most common endocrine tumor associated with CNC and is present in 25% of cases.

More than 75% of men with CNC may have large-cell calcifying Sertoli cell tumors of the testicles (LCCSCT). These tumors are usually bilateral and multifocal.

Furthermore, more than 75% of patients with CNC have multiple thyroid nodules, most of which are related to follicular adenomas. Psammomatous melanoma schwannoma, a benign neoplastic lesion derived from schwann cells, is observed in 10% of CNC patients at about 20 years of age.

With respect to pituitary lesions, more than 75% of patients with CNC show an asymptomatic increase in growth hormone (GH), insulin growth factor type 1 or prolactin; however, a detectable tumor is observed in less than 10% of cases.

21.4. Genetics

In 70% of cases, the CNC appears as an autosomal dominant hereditary trait with complete penetrance, while in the remaining cases the complex manifests sporadically. The prevalence of CNC is unclear due to the low frequency of the disorder.

Mutations that inactivate the PRKAR1A gene are responsible for the phenotypic manifestations of CNC in more than 70% of cases and are classified as category 1 (CNC 1). More than 125 different mutations in the PRKAR1A gene have been described to date in more than 400 families of different ethnic origins with CNC. Most of the mutations are of the nonsense type.

In addition, in patients with unmodified clinical criteria for prostate cancer without a PRKAR1A gene mutation, a second CNC locus has been identified, corresponding to a 10 Mb region of chromosome 2p16, found by linkage analysis. Tumors in patients with CNC have revealed changes in the copy number of this region; this group is referred to as CNC type 2. The affected genes at this site have not yet been identified. However, since the CNC1 and CNC2 phenotypes are not significantly different, it has been suggested that the genes involved may also be involved in the same molecular pathway.

Germline duplication of PRKACA is linked to bilateral adrenal-linked hyperplasia, in its different presentations, while somatic mutations in the same gene result in unilateral cortisol-producing adenomas of the adrenal gland.

In patients with an isolated presentation of PPNAD, the germline presence of copy number gains (duplication) of the chromosome 19 genomic region, which includes the PRKACA gene, has been confirmed.

21.5. Monitoring

Clinical evaluation of all manifestations of CNC should be performed at least once a year in all patients and should begin in infancy. Monitoring is different depending on the patients' stage of development. We distinguish between the prepubescent and postpubescent stages.

21.5.1. *Screening of prepubescent children*

Cardiac ultrasound should be started within the first six months and performed at least once a year thereafter. In patients with a history of cardiac myxoma, screening should be more frequent, optimally every six months.

Screening for other manifestations should be performed in patients under five years of age. Testicular ultrasound is recommended at the initial assessment. If microcalcifications are present, it should be repeated once a year.

Growth rate should be monitored as pediatric patients with CNC may have developmental delays, which may result from various CNC components, such as Cushing's syndrome due to PPNAD or liver damage.

21.5.2. *Annual screening of children and postpubescent adults*

The monitoring program combines both biochemical analyses and medical imaging techniques as follows:

– PPNAD by measurement of urinary free cortisol;

– acromegaly by measuring serum levels of GH, prolactin (PRL) and insulin-like growth factor I (IGF I);

– thyroid nodules by ultrasound as needed;

– LCCSCT in men by testicular ultrasound, especially when small calcifications are found;

– premenstrual syndrome with MRI of the spine once as a reference and then when clinical signs suggest the presence of a tumor;

– both breast myxomas and ductal adenomas in women should be screened and followed up as part of breast cancer screening, including self-screening palpation, clinical evaluation, mammography and ultrasound. If detected, MRI of the breast may be more sensitive in mapping lesions;

– ovarian lesions by transabdominal ultrasound at first assessment. The test should be repeated because of the low risk of ovarian malignancy.

DEFINITION.– Acromegaly *is a disorder that results from an excess of GH after the growth plates have closed. The initial symptom is usually an enlargement of the hands and feet, as well as an enlargement of the forehead, jaw and nose.*

22

Hematological Malignancies

22.1. Introduction

Inherited cancer syndromes associated with leukemia, such as familial myelodysplastic syndromes (MDSs) and acute myeloid leukemia (AML) syndromes, were once considered rare, but are actually more common than expected. The number of genes known to be involved in inherited MDS/AML has recently increased with the advancement of genomic sequencing technologies and the known inherited cancer syndromes associated with leukemia represent more than 60 different genes.

Cancer predisposition disorders may present with bone marrow failure (BMF), hematological malignancy, MDS or non-hematological manifestations, many of which overlap and may complicate diagnosis.

Leukemia predisposition syndromes include Fanconi anemia, Diamond–Blackfan anemia (DBA), Shwachman–Diamond syndrome (SDS), and dyskeratosis congenita (DC) and telomere biology disorders. In addition to the BMF syndromes mentioned above, other predisposition disorders for myeloid leukemia include those caused by germline mutations in the following genes: ANKRD26, CEBPA, DDX41, ELANE, ETV6, GATA2, HAX1, RUNX1, SAMD9, SAMD9L and SRP72. An inherited predisposition to lymphoid malignancies has also been described, including those caused by germline mutations in the genes ETV6, PAX5 and TP53. Leukemias caused by familial mutations in the IKZF1 gene are also likely to become a distinct syndrome.

There are different ways of classifying these different syndromes. Below, these syndromes have been divided into the following eight main categories based on clinical features, biological functions and affected pathways: (1) genetic instability/DNA repair syndromes; (2) RAS pathway dysfunction; (3) spinal cord insufficiency syndromes; (4) telomeropathies; (5) immunodeficiency; (6) transcription factor abnormalities; (7) pure familial leukemia; and (8) aneuploidy.

Some of these syndromes have been described in other sections of this book and will not be detailed here: Li–Fraumeni syndrome (LFS), RASopathies, constitutional mismatch repair-deficiency (CMMRD) syndrome, Werner syndrome, Bloom syndrome, Fanconi anemia, ataxia–telangiectasia, Noonan syndrome and neurofibromatosis type 1 (NF1).

22.2. Gene

1) Genetic instability/DNA repair:

- the most representative syndrome in this category is LFS, caused by the TP53 mutation;

- the recently described CMMRD syndrome is caused by biallelic (homozygous) alterations in the MMR genes, including MLH1, MSH2, MSH6 and PMS2;

- the category DNA repair deficiency/genetic instability also includes Werner syndrome (WRN), Rothmund–Thomson syndrome (RECQL4), Bloom syndrome (BLM), Fanconi anemia (FANC genes), ataxia–telangiectasia (ATM) and Nijmegen breakage syndrome (NBS1).

2) RAS pathway dysfunction: includes Noonan syndrome (PTPN11, K-RAS, N-RAS, etc.), CBL syndrome (CBL) and NF1.

3) Spinal cord insufficiency syndromes: these syndromes have numerous mutated genes, including DBA, SDS, familial aplastic anemia with SRP72 mutation, congenital amegalocytic thrombocytopenia (CAMT) syndrome, thrombocytopenia and absent radii (TAR), thrombocytopenia with ANKRD26 mutation and Kostmann syndrome. Recently, the RPS29, RPS27 and RPL27 genes have been implicated in DBA by whole exome sequencing.

4 and 5) Telomeropathies and immunodeficiency: DC is the representative disease of telomeropathies caused by a dysfunction of TERT and TERC, leading to abnormal maintenance of the telomeres. Until now, ACD, CTC1, DKC1, NHP2, NOP10, PARN, RTEL1, TERC, TERT, TINF2 and WRAP53 are the genes in which pathogenic variants are known to be responsible for DC formation.

6) Transcription factor abnormalities: inherited syndromes in this category are caused by mutations in genes encoding hematopoietic transcription factors. Alterations in associated genes (RUNX1, GATA2, PAX5, SH2B3 and ETV6) are also known to occur in *de novo* or sporadic leukemia cells.

7) Pure familial leukemia: the first gene involved in this category, CEBPA, was identified a decade ago. There have been more genes in this category, illustrated by multiple autosomal dominant, highly penetrating inherited cancer syndromes resulting from germline mutations in GATA2, DDX41 ATG2B and GSKIP. Familial chromosome 7 mosaic monosomy also falls into this category.

8) Aneuploidy: in addition to somatic aneuploidies, constitutional aneuploidies are also associated with the risk of specific hematological malignancies. Trisomy 21 and trisomy 8 are representatives of constitutional aneuploidies of the hereditary cancer syndrome associated with leukemia.

22.3. Tumors

A summarized description of the pathologies is as follows (for details, see the respective chapters of the different syndromes):

1) pediatric hematological malignancies, including ALL and AML; BMF (often occurs in childhood) leads to leukemia and MDS;

2) juvenile myelomonocytic leukemia (JMML) is a unique hematopoietic childhood disorder caused by excessive proliferation of cells from monocytic and granulocytic cell lines;

3) these spinal cord insufficiency syndromes are considered to be a risk factor for clonal evolution. In these syndromes, MDS and AML appear to be the most common hematological malignancies with risks ranging from 5–25%;

4 and 5) patients with DC are at increased risk of BMF, MDS or AML and solid tumors (usually squamous cell carcinoma of the head and neck or anogenital cancer and pulmonary fibrosis);

6) hereditary or sporadic mutations in the GATA2 gene induce MonoMAC syndrome (monocytopenia with atypical mycobacterial infection), DCML deficiency (loss of dendritic cells, monocytes, natural killer cells and B lymphoid cells), Emberger syndrome (lymphedema with MDS) and familial AML/MDS. More than half of patients with GATA2 deficiency develop MDS, most of whom will develop adverse chromosomal abnormalities and eventually progress to AML;

7) neoplasia in this category is exclusively leukemia;

8) constitutional trisomy 8 is less frequent than trisomy 21 and can be seen mainly as a mosaic in the blood or in the skin. Trisomy 8 is the most common cytogenetic abnormality among AMLs and MDSs, with incidences of 6% and 11%, respectively. Down syndrome (DS) results from trisomy 21 and occurs in 1 in 700–1,000 births. Patients with DS have a 10- to 20-fold increased risk of acute leukemia. The greatest increase in incidence in children with DS is related to acute megakaryoblastic leukemia (AMKL). It is estimated that the relative risk of developing AMKL is 500 times higher in children with DS than in the general population.

22.4. Genetics

Most of these syndromes are autosomal dominantly inherited, except for some types of DBA (GATA1 and TSR2) that are X-linked. However, CMMRD, Fanconi (except FANCR/RAD51 which is autosomal dominant and FANCB which is X-linked) and SDS demonstrate homozygous recessive transmission.

For DC, the types related to TERC, TINF2, NAF1 and STN1 are autosomal dominant; the types related to NOLA3/NOP10, NOLA2/NHP2, WRAP53/TCAB1 and CTC1 are autosomal recessive; the types linked to TERT, RTEL1, ACD/TPP1 and PARN are transmitted both autosomal recessively and autosomal dominantly and finally those linked to DKC1 are X-linked.

22.5. Monitoring

Careful monitoring for any signs or symptoms related to leukemia has been proposed for the management of these syndromes.

Patients with these hereditary syndromes are probably not as rare as previously thought. Most of these patients with leukemia should be treated with chemotherapy and/or allogeneic hematopoietic stem cell transplantation (HSCT), and should also be treated for their own hereditary syndromes because of their fragility. These problems become particularly important when planning HSCT, as patients with some of these syndromes are also at increased risk of developing complications during treatment.

DEFINITION.– *An* allograft *is a transplant of an organ, tissue or cells from one individual to another individual of the same species that is not an identical twin.*

Since JMML patients with CBL mutations and some of those with NRAS mutations may have spontaneous resolution of hematological abnormalities, the decision to perform HSCT in these patients should be weighed carefully.

These genetic abnormalities are also encountered as frequent somatic mutations in MDS/AML. Therefore, it is important to distinguish between somatic and germline mutations when evaluating syndromes associated with germline changes in these genes. For this reason, physicians need to be aware of these inherited predisposition syndromes and examine all clinical symptoms as well as the detailed family history of patients. The identification of these syndromes is a crucial step for individualized follow-up and treatment.

23

Familial Pituitary Adenomas

23.1. Introduction

Pituitary adenomas occur in about one in a thousand cases in the general population. Of these, about 95% are sporadic and occur without a recognized familial or hereditary cause. In 5% of pituitary adenomas, a number of inheritable genetic conditions have been identified at the germline level.

These genetic or genomic disorders may be limited to *familial isolated pituitary* adenomas (FIPA) or associated with a risk of disease of other organs in the context of syndromic endocrine neoplasia (MEN1, MEN4, hereditary pheochromocytomas and paragangliomas and CNC). The syndromic forms MEN1, MEN4, hereditary pheochromocytomas and paragangliomas and CNC have been discussed in other chapters of this book. In this chapter, we will limit ourselves to FIPA.

FIPA is characterized by the presence of both acromegaly and other pituitary adenomas in a familial framework, excluding the involvement of MEN1 and other syndromic forms. Thus, FIPA is defined as the presence of two or more related individuals with pituitary adenomas within the same family in the absence of known syndromic conditions such as MEN1 and CNC.

Two genetic causes of FIPA have been identified to date and account for approximately 20% of these patients. First, germline mutations in the AIP gene have been associated with predisposition to pituitary adenoma; the second genetic cause relates to microduplication on the Xq26.3 chromosome involving the GPR101 gene (X-linked male acrogigantic (X-LAG) syndrome).

23.2. Gene

The AIP (aryl hydrocarbon receptor (AHR)-interacting protein) gene, located on chromosome 11q13, codes for an intracellular protein of 330 amino acids (usually cytosolic), which is ubiquitously expressed in healthy tissues. AIP interacts with multiple partners, including the AHR, which acts as a dioxin receptor and mediates xenobiotic responses. In addition, AIP has a number of important interactions that may contribute to its tumorigenic role in the pituitary gland, including chaperones, phosphodiesterases, the α_i subunit of protein G and the zinc finger protein ZAC1 (also known as PLAGL1).

GPR101, an orphan G-protein coupled receptor, plays a central role in X-LAG syndrome. GPR101 is highly overexpressed in resected pituitary tissue in patients with X-LAG syndrome (an increase of several hundred to thousands of times). In addition, GPR101 is normally expressed in a very restricted set of tissues in humans, including the hypothalamus. GPR101 variants including missense change p.E308D may alter GH secretion in *in vitro* pituitary tumor models and these changes may contribute to tumorigenesis.

23.3. Tumors

FIPA patients have a younger age of onset than patients with sporadic pituitary adenomas (approximately five years earlier).

Somatotrophinomas account for approximately 70% of pituitary adenomas in patients with AIP mutations. Mixed or co-secreting GH/prolactin adenomas, prolactinomas or rare non-functional tumors, and very rarely Cushing's disease have also been described. Patients with AIP-related mutations are more frequently male (55–60%), especially in FIPA families with AIP mutations.

The overwhelming majority of patients with AIP-related pituitary adenomas already have a macroadenoma at the time of diagnosis. Macroadenomas have been shown to be present in almost 90% of cases at diagnosis, with 60–80% having extrasellar extension and 56% being invasive.

Acromegaly patients with AIP mutations are significantly younger at diagnosis and early symptoms have a larger maximum tumor diameter, higher GH levels at diagnosis and more frequently co-secreted prolactin.

X-LAG syndrome is characterized by a mixture of adenomas secreting GH and prolactin and/or hyperplasia. At diagnosis, the tumor is usually a macroadenoma. The resected pituitary tissue in some patients with X-LAG syndrome has extensive pituitary hyperplasia with formation of microadenomas in the hyperplastic tissue, suggesting that X-LAG pituitary pathology begins with a hyperplastic state, followed by the formation of adenomas. Pituitary tumors of X-LAG syndrome are highly functional with very high levels of GH, IGF-1 and usually prolactin.

23.4. Genetics

The mode of transmission of FIPA related to deleterious variations in the AIP gene is autosomal dominant with incomplete penetrance (of the order of 20%). The low penetrance rate may lead to confusion with sporadic cases, however true cases of *de novo* AIP mutations occurring sporadically are rarely encountered.

In a Finnish cohort, most members shared an identical truncation mutation of AIP, p.Q14X, which is almost exclusively limited to patients of Finnish origin. In an Italian cohort, another truncating mutation, p.R304X, was found. Since then, this mutation has proved to be the most frequently identified and appears separately in populations worldwide. Since then, other founder mutations associated with p.R304X have been noted, including an extended group linked to a founder mutation in Ireland. The arginine residue at position 304 is a hotspot that may also lead to a missense mutation (p.R304Q). A number of other common recurrent AIP mutations have been identified in families around the world, including p.R271W and p.R81X.

In the case of microduplication on chromosome Xq26.3 involving the GPR101 gene, duplication may occur either constitutionally in families, sporadically or as a mosaic in affected patients. Patients with sporadic X-LAG syndrome are somatic mosaics for Xq26.3 duplication. Sporadic male patients have dramatic pituitary giantism despite the fact that only 16–50% of the cells are positive for duplication (compared to constitutional duplication in women).

23.5. Monitoring

Screening for pituitary adenoma in children and adolescents should include screening for mutations in both the AIP and MEN1 genes, both of which are increasingly common in young people.

Pediatric patients with AIP mutations are predominantly somatotrophinoma patients, while less than 1.5% of pediatric Cushing's disease patients have AIP mutations.

Baseline X-ray imaging studies should be performed on newly identified mutation carriers, preferably a contrast-enhanced pituitary magnetic resonance imaging (MRI). In AIP mutation carriers with no evidence of pituitary tumor after baseline studies, clinical follow-up and hormone testing should be performed.

The interval between follow-up visits depends on the age of the patient and should be prioritized during the period when most AIP-related pituitary adenomas are expected (childhood to early adulthood).

Elderly carriers of AIP mutations who are unaffected (those over 40 years of age) may never develop pituitary adenoma, and follow-up after initial baseline assessments should take this into account to avoid unnecessarily repeated testing. An important issue is the confounding effect of accidental pituitary adenomas diagnosed by MRI when screening for carriers of the AIP mutation.

Patients with signs or symptoms of acromegaly should first be assessed with serum IGF-1. IGF-1 levels correlate well with GH activity. If serum IGF-1 levels are increased, a growth hormone suppression test should be performed with an oral glucose loading test.

MRI imaging of the pituitary gland should be performed, if not contraindicated, to assess the size, location and extent of parasellar involvement. Patients with symptoms of acromegaly should also be evaluated for possible co-morbidities of sleep apnea, diabetes mellitus, hypertension and osteoarthritis.

The morbidity and mortality associated with acromegaly is increased due to the effects of increased IGF-1 levels on the target organ, including the consequences on tumor mass and associated co-morbidities.

The main treatment strategy is to normalize GH and IGF-1 levels, reduce symptoms and control tumor mass. If the tumor is deemed resectable, transphenoidal resection is the most common treatment method. Experienced surgeons can improve clinical outcomes for more than 40% of macroadenomas and more than 85% of microadenomas.

DEFINITION.– Transphenoidal resection *is a type of surgery in which instruments are inserted through the nose and sphenoid sinus (a hollow space in a bone in the nose) to remove tumors in or near the pituitary gland. The pituitary gland is a pea-sized organ located at the base of the brain above the back of the nose.*

Patients with large tumors that are difficult to resect may require surgery and/or additional medical treatment. Persistence of disease despite surgery may require the use of somatostatin receptor ligands (i.e. octreotide) and/or GH receptor antagonists. In addition, radiotherapy should be considered in patients who cannot tolerate medical treatment or for whom no medication is available.

24

Bloom Syndrome

24.1. Introduction

Bloom syndrome (BS) is an autosomal recessive disorder characterized by prenatal and postnatal growth delay, photosensitive skin changes (erythematous skin lesions of the face, "typically" a butterfly-shaped distribution around the nose), immune deficiency, insulin resistance and a significantly increased risk of early onset of cancer and development of multiple cancers. Mutations with loss of function in the BLM gene, which codes for a RecQ helicase, cause BS. Cancer is the most common and serious medical complication in patients with BS and is the most common cause of death. Unlike many cancer predisposition syndromes that present a risk for one cancer or a small group of cancers, a wide variety of cancer types and anatomical localizations have been reported in patients with BS.

24.2. Gene

The BLM is the only gene known to cause the BS phenotype. The BLM gene is located on chromosome 15q26.1.

The BLM gene codes for a DNA helicase whose function is to facilitate DNA unfolding, an activity that uses the energy of ATP hydrolysis to move along the single-stranded DNA (ssDNA) and to break the hydrogen bonds that hold the two strands of DNA together. DNA helicases are involved in all DNA activities that require the opening of the duplex, including DNA replication, RNA transcription, homologous recombination and many other forms of DNA repair. The protein BLM has several different and important functions in maintaining genomic integrity.

Constitutional Oncogenetics,
Noureddine BOUKHATEM. © ISTE Ltd 2021.

24.3. Tumors

Leukemia and lymphoma are the most common type of cancer in patients with BS. The mean age of diagnosis for acute myelocytic leukemia (AML) is 18 years (range 2–47 years) and the mean age of diagnosis for acute lymphocytic leukemia (ALL) is 20 years (range 5–40 years). AML occurs about twice as often as ALL. Although both AML and ALL are associated with primary and secondary tumors, excess AML appears to be related to its occurrence following chemotherapy for a previous primary tumor, and when this occurs, the diagnosis of AML is usually preceded by a diagnosis of myelodysplastic syndrome.

The mean age of lymphomas at diagnosis is 22 years (4–49 years) and the types of lymphomas include B-cells (including Burkitt lymphoma) and T cells, but not Hodgkin's lymphoma. In about 75% of cases, lymphoma is the first tumor to occur and in about 25% of cases it is a second malignancy.

Among solid tumors, cancers of the digestive tract are the most common, particularly adenocarcinomas of the upper and lower digestive tracts. Squamous cell carcinomas of the head and neck have also been frequently diagnosed.

In addition to common malignancies, patients with BS also have an excess of rare cancers, particularly Wilms' tumor, which has been diagnosed in eight patients at an average age of three years. All classes of solid tumors have a mean age at diagnosis in patients with BS, significantly earlier than the same tumors in the general population.

24.4. Genetics

BS is an autosomal recessive rare disease caused by mutations in the BLM gene. It occurs more frequently in the Ashkenazi Jewish population compared to other populations due to a founder effect.

The frequency of carriers of a common pathogenic variant (blm^{Ash}) was found to be one in 107 in a cohort of 1,491 persons of Ashkenazi Jewish origin. The prevalence of the disease in this population is estimated to be approximately 1 in 48,000. In non-Jewish populations, the prevalence is not known. BS is very rare with less than 300 documented cases since it was first described in 1954.

Recent studies have suggested that heterozygotes of a pathogenic variant of the BLM, although otherwise healthy, have an increased risk of developing cancer. Heterozygotes of genes important in maintaining genomic integrity may be at increased risk of cancer due to reduced efficiency of DNA repair in heterozygous cells or loss of the normal allele resulting in the emergence of a somatic clone with a very high mutation rate.

24.5. Monitoring

Since BS is rare, there are no factual guidelines for management. Knowledge of the associated medical problems, however, provides a rational basis for monitoring and treatment. Although patients with BS have many medical and health problems, the main concerns remain skin abnormalities, growth and nutritional problems, endocrinological abnormalities and cancer risk.

A cancer monitoring program is important for patients with BS, but at this time there is no consensus on the most effective approach. Since there is no clear evidence that early detection of leukemia improves outcomes, monitoring such as routine complete blood counts is not recommended. Observation of all subjects with BS for characteristic signs and symptoms such as malaise, fever, night sweats, or lymphadenopathy should be immediately brought to the attention of a physician for further assessment.

Unintentional weight loss should also be considered as a possible symptom of malignancy. The increased risk of gastrointestinal cancers, especially of the colon, deserves special attention. Warning signs should be looked for in dark stools, rectal bleeding or other gastrointestinal problems.

A colonoscopy screening should therefore be considered at 16 years of age and performed regularly, although the appropriate interval is not known. Unfortunately, it is not possible to create a screening protocol for all types of cancer observed in patients with BS. A general state of vigilance and early medical attention is therefore warranted for any potential signs of malignancy, including abnormal or nodule growth, chronic pain or fatigue.

25

Werner Syndrome

25.1. Introduction

Werner syndrome (WS) is a rare genetic disorder with clinical signs of accelerated ageing. WS patients between the ages of 20 and 30 have characteristics similar, but not identical, to those of normal elderly people, including skin atrophy, aging and hair loss, wrinkles, fat loss, cataracts, atherosclerosis and diabetes. WS is caused by null mutations in the WRN gene, which codes for a member of the DNA helicase family: RecQ.

25.2. Gene

The WRN locus is located on chromosome 8p12, consists of 34 coding exons and has a size of 140 kb. The encoded WRN protein is a multifunctional nuclear protein of 1,432 amino acids and 160 kDa with a 3' → 5' exonuclease domain in its N-terminal region, an ATP-dependent 3' → 5' helicase in its central region and a nuclear localization signal in its C-terminal region. There are two other consensus domains: the conserved helicase region RecQ (RQC) and the conserved helicase region, RNaseD C-terminal (HRDC).

WRN is part of the RecQ helicase protein family and has the particularity of possessing both helicase and exonuclease domains. WRN also has strand renaturation activity, but its role *in vivo* remains unclear.

WRN is mainly localized in the nucleolus and then moves to DSBs (double-strand break DNA) when they appear. In response to DNA damage, WRN interacts with several proteins that are involved in the repair of DNA by homologous recombination (HR), non-homologous end joining (NHEJ) and single strand renaturation.

Several data sources suggest that telomere dysfunction contributes to WS pathology. WRN-deficient cells undergo early replicative senescence and telomere loss and chromosomal rearrangements.

WRN acts at the telomeres to promote replication and suppress recombination. Cells use telomerase, which are reverse transcriptases with an RNA component, Terc, to replicate and elongate telomeres. WRN helicase activity is thought to contribute to telomere replication by resolving or dissolving complex DNA structures found at telomeres such as T-loops, D-loops and G-quartets (G4).

25.3. Tumors

Systematic reviews of cancers in WS patients have revealed a much higher incidence of sarcoma than expected for a control cohort of the same age. The most common neoplasms in WS patients are follicular carcinomas of the thyroid, followed by malignant melanoma, meningioma, soft tissue sarcomas, primary bone tumors and leukemia/myelodysplasia. The risk of these tumors varies, and it is 2–60 times higher than that of controls in the general population. Furthermore, the reason why patients with WS are predisposed to non-epithelial malignancies remains to be determined.

25.4. Genetics

The overall incidence is estimated at between 1/1,000,000 and 1/10,000,000. However, the incidence is higher in Japan, with one in 100,000 births. The mode of transmission of WS is autosomal recessive.

WS is caused by a loss of homozygous or heterozygous composite function of the WRN. WRN is the only known gene in which mutations cause classical WS, and WS is the only known genetic disorder caused by null mutations in the WRN gene.

More than 70 different mutations have been identified. A majority of the mutations are stop codons, small indels or splice mutations that cause truncations with loss of the nuclear localization signal at the C-terminal end of the WRN protein and/or promote the termination of translation of mutant mRNA induced by nonsense codons. Two amino acid substitution mutations in the exonuclease domain, p.Lys125Asn and Lys135Glu, render the WRN protein unstable and are also functionally null mutations.

25.5. Monitoring

Early diagnosis of WS is important to reduce complications and prolong life. Those affected should be examined regularly for secondary metabolic disorders, atherosclerosis, cardiac/brain disorders and associated cancers.

Clinical management has focused on the treatment of manifestations, prevention of secondary complications and screening for acquired diseases common to WS. The treatment of WS patients is similar to that of the general population, with the exception of neoplasia, where the use of DNA-damaging chemotherapeutic agents can be modified to reflect the sensitivity of WS cells to several classes of chemotherapeutic agents.

Appendix

Summary of the Book

COMMENT ON TABLE A.1.– *Table legend:*

– 1: in an asymptomatic person (free of neoplasia);

– 2: as genetic testing allows for a more accurate diagnosis of the disease;

– 3: mainly malignant tumors;

– 4: the risk of cancer is nil before adulthood, but benign tumors appear very early in childhood and may justify undertaking the test in childhood;

– 5: AD: autosomal dominant;

– 6: AR: autosomal recessive;

– 7: risk in the event of a deleterious mutation of the gene(s) in question. Nevertheless, it should be noted that a high risk does not necessarily mean that the type of cancer is frequent.

Gene	Syndrome	Mode of transmission	Tumors/organs[3]	Magnitude of absolute risk	Evidence level	Age for the predictive test[1]	Chapter
BRCA1	HBOC: Hereditary breast and ovarian cancer	AD[5]	Breast	High for females, very low for males	Sufficient	Adult (preferably after 25 years of age)	1
			Ovary, fallopian tubes, peritoneum	High	Sufficient		
			Prostate	Not determined	Insufficient		
			Pancreas	Very low	Insufficient		
BRCA2	HBOC	AD	Breast	High for females, very low for males	Sufficient	Adult (preferably after 25 years of age)	1
			Ovary, fallopian tubes, peritoneum	Moderate	Sufficient		
			Prostate	High	Sufficient		
			Pancreas	Low	Sufficient		
CHEK2	HBOC	AD	Breast	Moderate	Sufficient	Adult (preferably after 25 years of age)	1

Gene	Syndrome	Mode of transmission	Tumors/organs[3]	Magnitude of absolute risk	Evidence level	Age for the predictive test[1]	Chap.
PALB2	HBOC	AD	Breast	High	Sufficient	Adult (preferably after 25 years of age)	1
NBN	HBOC	AD	Breast	Low	Insufficient	Not determined	1
			Ovary	Low	Insufficient		
BARD1	HBOC	AD	Breast	Low	Insufficient	Not determined	1
BRIP1	HBOC	AD	Ovary, fallopian tubes, peritoneum	Low	Sufficient	Adult (preferably after 25 years of age)	1
RAD51C	HBOC	AD	Ovary, fallopian tubes, peritoneum	Moderate	Sufficient	Adult (preferably after 25 years of age)	1
RAD51D	HBOC	AD	Ovary, fallopian tubes, peritoneum	Moderate	Sufficient	Adult (preferably after 25 years of age)	1

Gene	Syndrome	Mode of transmission	Tumors/organs[3]	Magnitude of absolute risk	Evidence level	Age for the predictive test[1]	Chap.
ATM	Ataxia–telangiectasia	AR[6]	Breast	Moderate, but high for the V2424G mutation.	Sufficient	Childhood and according to mutation and family history	1 and 12
			Lymphoid malignancies	High	Sufficient		
			Epithelial cancers	Low	Sufficient		
MLH1 MSH2 MSH6 PMS2 EPCAM	LS: Lynch syndrome	AD	Colorectal and endometrial cancer mainly in addition to gastrointestinal cancers, genitourinary tract cancers and breast cancer more rarely	Very high for colorectal, high for endometrial, low for gastrointestinal, breast and ovarian and very low for pancreas, urinary tract and prostate.	Sufficient	Adulthood (assessment according to family history)	2

Gene	Syndrome	Mode of transmission	Tumors/organs[3]	Magnitude of absolute risk	Evidence level	Age for the predictive test[1]	Chap.
MLH1 MSH2 MSH6 PMS2	MTS: Muir–Torre syndrome	AD or AR	Visceral LS spectrum malignancy and skin neoplasia	Very low	Sufficient	Adulthood (assessment according to family history)	2
MLH1 MSH2 MSH6 PMS2	TS: Turcot syndrome	AD	Co-occurrence of a brain tumor (glioma/glioblastoma) with a colorectal tumor	Low	Sufficient	Adulthood (assessment according to family history)	2
APC			Co-occurrence of a brain tumor (medulloblastoma) with a colorectal tumor				
MLH1 MSH2 MSH6 PMS2	CMMR-D: Constitutional MMR deficiencies	AR	LS spectrum in addition to astrocytoma	High	Sufficient	Early childhood, around 5 years old	2

Gene	Syndrome	Mode of transmission	Tumors/organs[3]	Magnitude of absolute risk	Evidence level	Age for the predictive test[1]	Chap.
APC	FAP: Familial adenomatous polyposis	AD	CRC: Colorectal	Very high	Sufficient	Variable according to the degree of polyposis (from ten years old)	4
	AFAP: Attenuated FAP					Adulthood	
	TS		CRC + brain tumor (medulloblastoma)	Very high for CRC and low for medulloblastoma			
MUTYH	MAP: Polyposis associated with MUTYH	AR	CRC + duodenum, ovary, bladder and skin	High for CRC and low for others	Sufficient for CRC	Adulthood	4
NTHL1	NAP: Polyposis associated with NTHL1	AR	CRC + endometrium, duodenum, skin, breast and pancreas	High for CRC and low for others	Sufficient for CRC	Adulthood	4
POLE POLD1	PPAP: Polyposis associated with polymerase proofreading activity	AD	CRC + pancreas, ovaries, small intestine, endometrium and brain	High for CRC and low for others	Sufficient for CRC	Adulthood	4

Gene	Syndrome	Mode of transmission	Tumors/organs[3]	Magnitude of absolute risk	Evidence level	Age for the predictive test[1]	Chap.
NF1	Neurofibromatosis 1	AD	Malignant tumors of the peripheral nerve sheath	High	Sufficient	Childhood, adolescence	3
			Optic nerve gliomas and brain tumors	Low	Sufficient		
			Breast	Very low			
			Leukemia (especially juvenile chronic myeloid leukemia)	Very low			
NF2	Neurofibromatosis 2	AD	Vestibular schwannomas, intracranial meningiomas and spinal tumors	Very high	Sufficient	From birth	3
LZTR1 SMARCB1	Schwannomatosis	AD	Schwannomas of the spinal cord, chest wall and subcutaneous regions	Very high	Sufficient	Adulthood	3

Gene	Syndrome	Mode of transmission	Tumors/organs[3]	Magnitude of absolute risk	Evidence level	Age for the predictive test[1]	Chap.
MEN1	Multiple endocrine neoplasia type 1	AD	Mainly (neuro) endocrine, parathyroid, pituitary and pancreatic tumors; less frequently adrenocortical and carcinoid tumors	Very high	Sufficient	Five years	5
RET	Multiple endocrine neoplasia type 2/MEN2A	AD	MTC: medullary thyroid carcinoma, associated with pheochromocytoma and/or multiple tumors of the parathyroid glands	Very high	Sufficient	Childhood	5
	Multiple endocrine neoplasia type 2/MEN2B	AD	MTC + pheochromocytoma, without hyperparathyroidism	Very high	Sufficient	Childhood	5

Gene	Syndrome	Mode of transmission	Tumors/organs[3]	Magnitude of absolute risk	Evidence level	Age for the predictive test[1]	Chap.
	Multiple endocrine neoplasia type 2/FMTC: Familial MTC	AD	MTC with a very low incidence of other clinical manifestations of MEN2A	Very high		Childhood	5
CDKN1B	Multiple endocrine neoplasia type 4	AD	Pituitary neuroendocrine tumor and PitNET (somatotrophic, corticotropic and non-functional adenomas)	Very high	Sufficient	Adolescence	5
CDC73	HPT-JT: Hyperparathyroidism jaw tumor syndrome	AD	Parathyroid adenomas, maxillary or mandibular bone fibroids or infrequently parathyroid cancers and benign and malignant uterine tumors	Very high	Sufficient	Five years	5

Gene	Syndrome	Mode of transmission	Tumors/organs[3]	Magnitude of absolute risk	Evidence level	Age for the predictive test[1]	Chap.
SDHD	PGL1: Familial inherited PGL syndrome type 1	AD modified by the original parent (paternal transmission)	Paraganglioma (PGL) of the head and neck with rare abdominal extra adrenal PGLs or pheochromocytomas; GIST: gastrointestinal stromal tumors; renal carcinomas	Very high	Sufficient	Six years	6
SDHAF2	PGL2: Familial inherited PGL syndrome type 2	AD modified by the original parent (paternal transmission)	PGL of the head and neck	Very high	Sufficient	Adulthood	6
SDHC	PGL3: Familial inherited PGL syndrome type 3	AD	PGL of the head and neck with rarely adrenal abdominal PGLs or pheochromocytomas; GIST: gastrointestinal stromal tumors; renal carcinomas	Very high	Sufficient	Adulthood	6

Gene	Syndrome	Mode of transmission	Tumors/organs[3]	Magnitude of absolute risk	Evidence level	Age for the predictive test[1]	Chap.
SDHB	PGL4: Familial inherited PGL syndrome type 4	AD	Extra adrenal PGL, rarely; GIST: gastrointestinal stromal tumors; renal carcinomas	Very high	Sufficient	Eight years	6
SDHA	PGL5: Familial inherited PGL syndrome type 5	AD	Pheochromocytoma or extra adrenal PGL	Very high	Sufficient	Eight years	6
MAX	Hereditary pheochromocytoma	AD modified by the original parent (paternal transmission)	Bilateral or multiple pheochromocytoma	Very high	Sufficient	Adulthood	6
TMEM127	Hereditary pheochromocytoma	AD	Pheochromocytoma mainly; extra adrenal PGL, including head and neck PGL less frequently	Very high	Sufficient	Adulthood	6

Gene	Syndrome	Mode of transmission	Tumors/organs[3]	Magnitude of absolute risk	Evidence level	Age for the predictive test[1]	Chap.
EPAS1 HIF2A EGLN1 EGLN2	Hereditary pheochromocytomas	AD	Multifocal PGL, PGL simultaneous with or after PCC	Very high	Sufficient	Eight years	6
FLCN	BHD: Birt–Hogg–Dubé syndrome	AD	Renal tumors: renal chromophobic carcinoma or hybrid oncocytic tumors (renal chromophobic carcinoma/renal oncocytoma)	Moderate	Sufficient	Adulthood	7
PTPN11 SOS1 RAF1 KRAS NRAS SHOC2 CBL	Noonan syndrome	AD	Myeloid, myogenic and neural tumors with rhabdomyosarcoma and neuroblastoma frequently observed in Costello and Noonan syndromes; very rare epithelial cancers and melanomas; myeloproliferative disorder (MPD) with malignant course in Noonan syndrome	Low	Sufficient	Childhood[2]	8

Gene	Syndrome	Mode of transmission	Tumors/organs[3]	Magnitude of absolute risk	Evidence level	Age for the predictive test[1]	Chap.
PTPN11 RAF1	MSML/LEOPARD: Noonan syndrome with multiple lentigines	AD	Myeloid, myogenic and neural tumors with frequently observed rhabdomyosarcoma and neuroblastoma in Costello and Noonan syndromes; very rare epithelial cancers and melanomas; myeloproliferative disorder (MPD) with malignant evolution in Noonan syndrome	Very low	Insufficient	Childhood[2]	8
RASA1	Capillary malformation–arteriovenous malformation	AD		Very low	Insufficient	Childhood[2]	8
HRAS	Costello's Syndrome	AD		Moderate	Sufficient	Childhood[2]	8
BRAF MAP2K1 MAP2K2 KRAS	Cardio-facio-cutaneous syndrome	AD		Very low	Insufficient	Childhood[2]	8
CDKN2A	FAMMM: Atypical familial multiple melanoma syndrome	AD	Melanomas, pancreas; neoplasms of the nervous system	High	Sufficient	Adulthood	9
CDK4				Low			

Gene	Syndrome	Mode of transmission	Tumors/organs[3]	Magnitude of absolute risk	Evidence level	Age for the predictive test[1]	Chap.
CDKN2A	MAS: Melanoma–astrocytoma syndrome	AD	Melanomas, astrocytomas	High	Sufficient	Adulthood	9
CDK4				Low			
BAP1	Familial malignant melanoma	AD	Melanomas; uveal melanomas (more frequently with BAP1 mutations); clear cell renal carcinomas; chronic lymphocytic leukemia and thyroid cancer (POT1)	Moderate	Sufficient	Adulthood	9
MITF							
POT1							
PTCH1	GS: Gorlin syndrome (nevoid basal cell carcinoma syndrome)	AD	Basal cell carcinoma; desmoplastic medulloblastoma, meningioma, rhabdomyosarcoma	High	Sufficient	Six years	10
SUFU							

Gene	Syndrome	Mode of transmission	Tumors/organs[3]	Magnitude of absolute risk	Evidence level	Age for the predictive test[1]	Chap.
TP53	LFS: Li–Fraumeni syndrome	AD	Breast cancer; soft tissue sarcomas and osteosarcomas; central nervous system tumors; adrenal cortical carcinoma and leukemia	Very high	Sufficient	Five years	11
CASR GNA11 AP2S1 GCM2	PHPT group: Primary hereditary hyperparathyroidism (including FIHPT, FHH and NSHPT)	AD	Parathyroid carcinoma	Low	Sufficient	Adulthood	13
PTEN	CS: Cowden syndrome	AD	Breast cancer, thyroid cancer, endometrial cancer, colorectal cancer, kidney cancer and melanoma	High	Sufficient	Adulthood, but childhood in cases of macrocephaly and neurodevelopmental disorder or hamartomatous polyps	14.1
	BRRS: Bannayan–Riley–Ruvalcaba syndrome	AD	Risk of malignancy similar to individuals with CS	High	Sufficient		

Gene	Syndrome	Mode of transmission	Tumors/organs[3]	Magnitude of absolute risk	Evidence level	Age for the predictive test[1]	Chap.
BMPR1A SMAD4	JPS: Juvenile polyposis syndrome	AD	Colorectal cancer or cancer of the upper gastrointestinal tract; more rarely, cancers of the pancreas, small intestine, duodenum and jejunum	High	Sufficient	15 years old	14.2
STK11 (LKB1)	PJS: Peutz–Jeghers syndrome	AD	Cancer of the gastrointestinal tract, including the esophagus, stomach, small intestine, colon and pancreas; more rarely breast cancer; associated cancers of the reproductive organs (in both sexes)	High	Sufficient	Ten years	14.3
FANCA	FA: Fanconi anemia	AR	Acute myeloid leukemia (AML), squamous cell carcinoma of the head and neck and squamous cell carcinoma of the vulva	High	Sufficient	Childhood[2]	15
FANCB		Recessive X linked					
FANCC BRCA2/FANCD1		AR					
FANCD2 FANCE		AR					

Gene	Syndrome	Mode of transmission	Tumors/organs[3]	Magnitude of absolute risk	Evidence level	Age for the predictive test[1]	Chap.
FANCF							
FANCG							
FANCI							
BRIP1/FANCJ							
FANCL		AR					
FANCM							
RAD51C/FANCO							
SLX4/FANCP	FA: Fanconi anemia		Acute myeloid leukemia (AML), squamous cell carcinoma of the head and neck and squamous cell carcinoma of the vulva	High	Sufficient	Childhood[2]	15
ERCC4/FANCQ							
RAD51/FANCR		AD					
BRCA1/FANCS							
UBE2T/FANCT							
XRCC2/FANCU		AR					
MAD2L2/REV7/FANCV							

Gene	Syndrome	Mode of transmission	Tumors/organs[3]	Magnitude of absolute risk	Evidence level	Age for the predictive test[1]	Chap.
CDH1	HDGC: Hereditary diffuse gastric cancer	AD	Gastric cancer (cancer of the stomach (signet ring) and lobular breast cancer)	High	Sufficient	Adulthood	16
VHL	VHLS: Von Hippel–Lindau syndrome	AD	Pancreatic neuroendocrine tumors, clear cell carcinomas, pheochromocytomas and paragangliomas	High	Sufficient	Adulthood[4]	17
XPA XPB (ERCC3) XPC XPD (ERCC2) XPE (DDB2) XPF (ERCC4) XPG (ERCC5) XPV (POLH)	XP: *Xeroderma pigmentosum*	AR	Malignant tumors of melanocytes and keratinocytes *in situ*, possibly several basal cell carcinomas and invasive squamous cell carcinomas and melanomas	High in the absence of UV protection	Sufficient	From birth	18

Gene	Syndrome	Mode of transmission	Tumors/organs[3]	Magnitude of absolute risk	Evidence level	Age for the predictive test[1]	Chap.
MET	HPRC: Hereditary papillary kidney cancer type 1	AD	Papillary tumors type 1 (very slow growing)	High	Sufficient	Adulthood	19
FH	HLRCC: HPRC type 2 or hereditary leiomyoma cancer and renal cell carcinoma	AD	Papillary kidney tumors type 2 (more aggressive); uterine and cutaneous leiomyomas (possible malignant transformation)	High	Sufficient	Adulthood	19
RB1	RB: Retinoblastoma	AD	Retinoblastoma; PNET: primary intracranial neuroectodermal tumor	Very high	Sufficient	From birth	20
PRKAR1A PRKACA PRKACB	NCC: Carney complex (Carney syndrome)	AD	Endocrine and non-endocrine multiple neoplasia (PPNAD); large-cell calcifying Sertoli cell tumors (LCCSCT); pituitary tumors; thyroid nodules and rarely ovarian malignancy	High	Sufficient	Childhood	21

<table>
<tr><th>Gene</th><th>Syndrome</th><th>Mode of transmission</th><th>Tumors/organs[3]</th><th>Magnitude of absolute risk</th><th>Evidence level</th><th>Age for the predictive test[1]</th><th>Chap.</th></tr>
<tr><td>ANKRD26</td><td rowspan="15">Hematological malignancies (hereditary MDS/AML)</td><td rowspan="5">AD</td><td rowspan="15">ALL, AML, MDS, juvenile myelomonocytic leukemia (JMML), MonoMAC (monocytopenia with atypical mycobacterial infection), acute megakaryoblastic leukemia (AMKL) and solid tumors (usually squamous cell carcinoma of the head and neck or anogenital cancer and pulmonary fibrosis)</td><td rowspan="15">High</td><td rowspan="15">Sufficient</td><td rowspan="15">Childhood in general</td><td rowspan="15">22</td></tr>
<tr><td>CEBPA</td></tr>
<tr><td>DDX41</td></tr>
<tr><td>ELANE</td></tr>
<tr><td>ETV6</td></tr>
<tr><td>GATA1</td><td>X-linked</td></tr>
<tr><td>GATA2</td><td rowspan="9">AD</td></tr>
<tr><td>HAX1</td></tr>
<tr><td>RUNX1</td></tr>
<tr><td>SAMD9</td></tr>
<tr><td>SAMD9L</td></tr>
<tr><td>SRP72</td></tr>
<tr><td>ETV6</td></tr>
<tr><td>PAX5</td></tr>
<tr><td>TP53</td></tr>
</table>

Gene	Syndrome	Mode of transmission	Tumors/organs[3]	Magnitude of absolute risk	Evidence level	Age for the predictive test[1]	Chap.
TSR2	/	X-linked	ALL, AML, MDS, juvenile myelomonocytic leukemia (JMML), MonoMAC (monocytopenia with atypical mycobacterial infection), acute megakaryoblastic leukemia (AMKL) and solid tumors (usually squamous cell carcinoma of the head and neck or anogenital cancer and pulmonary fibrosis).	High	/	/	/
DKC1		AD					
TERC							
TINF2							
NAF1							
STN1							
NOLA3/NOP10		AR					
NOLA2/NHP2							
WRAP53/TCAB1							
CTC1							
IKZF1		AD					
AIP GPR101	Familial isolated pituitary adenomas (FIPA)	AD	Mixed adenomas or co-secreting GH/prolactin, prolactinomas	Moderate	Sufficient	Childhood	23

Gene	Syndrome	Mode of transmission	Tumors/organs[3]	Magnitude of absolute risk	Evidence level	Age for the predictive test[1]	Chap.
BLM	BS: Bloom syndrome	AR	Leukemias (AML and ALL) and lymphomas; cancers of the digestive tract are the most common, especially adenocarcinomas of the upper and lower digestive tracts; squamous cell carcinomas of the head and neck; Wilms' tumor	High	Sufficient	Childhood	24
WRN	WS: Werner syndrome	AR	Sarcomas; follicular carcinomas of the thyroid, malignant melanoma, meningioma, soft tissue sarcomas, primary bone tumors and leukemia/myelodysplasia	High	Sufficient	Adulthood	25

References

Birt–Hogg–Dubé syndrome

Bock, K., Lohse, Z., Madsen, P.H., Hilberg, O. (2018). Birt-Hogg-Dubé syndrome: Spontaneous pneumothorax as a first symptom. Case reports, 2018:bcr-2017-219979.

Fibla Alfara, J.J., López-Rodó, L.M., Ferrández, H., Guirao, A. (2017). Recurrent spontaneous pneumothorax as a manifestation of Birt-Hogg-Dubé syndrome. *Arch. Bronco-neumol.*, 54(7), 8–9.

Ganeshan, D., Morani, A., Gautam, R., Choyke, P.L., Kundra, V. (2017). The ABCs of BHD: An in-depth review of Birt-Hogg-Dubé syndrome. *American Journal of Roentgenology*, 209(6), 1291–1296.

Geilswijk, M., Bendstrup, E., Madsen, M.G., Sommerlund, M., Skytte, A.-B. (2018). Childhood pneumothorax in Birt-Hogg-Dubé syndrome: A cohort study and review of the literature. *Molecular Genetics and Genomic Medicine*, 6, 332– 338.

Schmidt, L.S. and Linehan, W.M. (2018). FLCN: The causative gene for Birt-Hogg-Dubé syndrome. *Gene*, 640, 28–42.

Steinlein, O.K., Ertl-Wagner, B., Ruzicka, T., Sattler, E.C. (2018). Birt-Hogg-Dubé syndrome: An underdiagnosed genetic tumor syndrome. *JDDG*, 16(3), 278–283.

Tong, Y., Schneider, J.A., Coda, A.B., Hata, T.R., Cohen, P.R. (2018). Birt-Hogg-Dubé syndrome: A review of dermatological manifestations and other symptoms. *American Journal of Clinical Dermatology*, 19(1), 87–101.

Breast-ovarian cancer syndrome

Afghahi, A. and Kurian, A.W. (2017). The changing landscape of genetic testing for inherited breast cancer predisposition. *Curr. Treat. Options Oncol.*, 18(5), 27.

Al Bakir, M. and Gabra, H. (2014). The molecular genetics of hereditary and sporadic ovarian cancer: Implications for the future. *Br. Med. Bull.*, 112(1), 57–69.

Artosch, C.A.B., Larke, B.L.C., Osse, T.J.B. (2018). Gynaecological neoplasms in common familial syndromes (Lynch and HBOC). *Pathology*, 50(2), 222–237.

Beirne, J.P., Irwin, G.W., McIntosh, S.A., Harley, I.J.G., Harkin, D.P. (2015). The molecular and genetic basis of inherited cancer risk in gynaecology. *TOG*, 17(4), 233–241.

Buys, S.S., Sandbach, J.F., Gammon, A., Patel, G., Kidd, J.A. (2017). Study of over 35,000 women with breast cancer tested with a 25-gene panel of hereditary cancer genes. *Cancer*, 123(10), 1721–1730.

Daly, M.B., Pilarski, R., Berry, M., Buys, S.S., Farmer, M., Friedman, S., Garber, J.E., Kauff, N.D., Khan, S., Klein, C., Kohlmann, W., Kurian, A., Litton, J.K., Madlensky, L., Merajver, S.D., Offit, K., Pal, T., Reiser, G., Mahoney Shannon, K., Swisher, E., Vinayak, S., Voian, N.C., Weitzel, J.N., Wick, M.J.m Wiesner, G.L., Dwyer, M., Darlow, S. (2018). NCCN guidelines insights: Genetic/familial high-risk assessment: Breast and ovarian. *Journal of the National Comprehensive Cancer Network*, 15(1), 9–20.

Eccles, D.M., Mitchell, G., Monteiro, A.N.A., Schmutzler, R., Couch, F.J., Spurdle, A.B. Gómez-García, E.B. (2015). BRCA1 and BRCA2 genetic testing – Pitfalls and recommendations for managing variants of uncertain clinical significance. *Ann. Oncol.*, 26(10), 2057–2065.

Eccles, D.M., Balmaña, J., Clune, J., Ehlken, B., Gohlke, A., Hirst, C., Potter, D., Schroeder, C., Tyczynski, J.E., Gómez-García, E.B. (2016). Selecting patients with ovarian cancer for germline BRCA mutation testing: Findings from guidelines and a systematic literature review. *Adv. Ther.*, 33(2), 129–150.

Gevensleben, H., Bossung, V., Meindl, A., Wappenschmidt, B., de Gregorio, N., Osorio, A., Romero, A., Buettner, R., Markiefka, B., Schmutzler, R.K. (2014). Pathological features of breast and ovarian cancers in RAD51C germline mutation carriers. *Virchows Arch.*, 465(3), 365–369.

Giri, V.N., Knudsen, K.E., Kelly, W.K., Abida, W., Andriole, G.L., Bangma, C.H., Bekelman, J.E., Benson, M.C., Blanco, A., Burnett, A. (2017). Role of genetic testing for inherited prostate cancer risk: Philadelphia prostate cancer consensus conference. *Journal of Clinical Oncology*, 36(4), 414.

Goetsch, A.L., Kimelman, D., Woodruff, T.K. (2017). Hereditary gynecologic cancer predisposition syndromes. In *Fertility Preservation and Restoration for Patients with Complex Medical Conditions*, Goetsch, A.L., Kimelman, D., Woodruff, T.K. (eds). Springer, Berlin, 7–18.

Gupta, I., Burney, I., Al-Moundhri, M.S., Tamimi, Y. (2017). Molecular genetics complexity impeding research progress in breast and ovarian cancers. *Mol. Clin. Oncol.*, 7(1), 3–14.

Hall, M.J. (2018). Breast and ovarian cancer penetrance estimates derived from germline multiple-gene sequencing results in women. *JCO Precision Oncology*, 1, 1–12.

Hoang, L.N. and Gilks, B.C. (2017). Hereditary breast and ovarian cancer syndrome: Moving beyond BRCA1 and BRCA2. *Adv. Anat. Pathol.*, 25(2), 1–11.

Hoogerbrugge, N. and Jongmans, M.C.J. (2016). Finding all BRCA pathogenic mutation carriers: Best practice models. *European Journal of Human Genetics*, 24, S19–S26.

Imyanitov, E.N. (2013). Ovarian cancer genome. In *Ovarian Cancer*, Malek, A., Tchernitsa, O. (eds). Humana Press, Totowa.

Jones, M.R., Kamara, D., Karlan, B.Y., Pharoah, P.D.P, Gayther, S.A. (2017). Gynecologic oncology genetic epidemiology of ovarian cancer and prospects for polygenic risk prediction. *Gynecol. Oncol.*, 147, 705–713.

Katapodi, M.C., Viassolo, V., Caiata-Zufferey, M. (2017). Cancer predisposition cascade screening for hereditary breast/ovarian cancer and Lynch syndromes in Switzerland: Study protocol. *JMIR Res. Protoc.*, 6, 1–17.

Kobayashi, H., Ohno, S., Sasaki, Y., Matsuura, M. (2013). Hereditary breast and ovarian cancer susceptibility genes (review). *Oncology Reports*, 30(3), 1019–1029.

Lee, M.K., Gulsuner, S., Bernards, S.S., Casadei, S., Norquist, B.M., Harrell, M.I., Brady, M.F., Walsh, T., Yi, Q., Burger, R.A., Chan, J.K., Davidson, S.A., Mannel, R.S., DiSilvestro, P.A., Lankes, H.A., Ramirez, N.C., King, M.C., Swisher, E.M., Birrer, M.J. (2017). Inherited mutations in women with ovarian carcinoma. *JAMA Oncology*, 2(4), 482–490.

Lilyquist, J., LaDuca, H., Polley, E., Tippin Davis, B., Shimelis, H., Hu, C., Hart, S.N., Dolinsky, J.S., Couch, F.J., Goldgar, D.E. (2017). Frequency of mutations in a large series of clinically ascertained ovarian cancer cases tested on multi-gene panels compared to reference controls. *Gynecol. Oncol.*, 147(2), 375–380.

Nguyen, A., Plichta, J.K., Cintolo-Gonzalez, J., Kartal, K., Griffin, M.E., Hughes, K. (2018). Genetic risk prediction in breast cancer. In *Changing Paradigms in the Management of Breast Cancer*, Howard-McNatt, M. (ed.). Springer, Cham, 217–232.

Palacios, J. and Castilla, M.A. (2008). The molecular pathology of hereditary. *Pathobiology*, 75(2), 85–94.

Pearls, C. (2018). The genetics of triple-negative breast cancer. *Curr. Probl. Cancer*, 40(2–4), 33–40.

Ramus, S.J., Song, H., Dicks, E., Tyrer, J.P., Rosenthal, A.N., Intermaggio, M.P., Fraser, L., Gentry-Maharaj, A., Hayward, J. and Philpott, S. (2015). Germline mutations in the BRIP1, BARD1, PALB2, and NBN genes in women with ovarian cancer. *J. Natl. Cancer Inst.*, 107(7), 1–8.

Rosenthal, E.T., Bernhisel, R., Brown, K., Kidd, J., Manley, S. (2017). Clinical testing with a panel of 25 genes associated with increased cancer risk results in a significant increase in clinically significant findings across a broad range of cancer histories. *Cancer Genet.*, 219, 58–68.

Satoh, T., Takamatsu, K., Takeshima, N., Kobayashi, H. (2017). Final report of the Committee on Gynecologic Oncology, the Japan Society of Obstetrics and Gynecology, on a fact-finding questionnaire on the status of treatment of hereditary breast and ovarian cancer syndrome in Japan. *J. Obstet. Gynaecol. Res.*, 43(9), 1377–1380.

Schoolmeester, J.K., Moyer, A.M., Goodenberger, M.L., Keeney, G.L., Carter, J.M., Bakkum-Gamez, J.N. (2017). Pathologic findings in breast, fallopian tube, and ovary specimens in non-BRCA hereditary breast and/or ovarian cancer syndromes: A study of 18 patients with deleterious germline mutations in RAD51C, BARD1, BRIP1, PALB2, MUTYH, or CHEK2. *Hum. Pathol.*, 70, 14–26.

Shieh, Y., Eklund, M., Madlensky, L., Sawyer, S.D., Thompson, C.K., Fiscalini, A.S., Ziv, E., van't Veer, L.J., Esserman, L., Tice, J.A. (2018). Breast cancer screening in the precision medicine era: Risk-based screening in a population-based trial. *Journal of the National Cancer Institute*, 109(5), 1–8.

Taylor, A., Brady, A.F., Frayling, I.M., Hanson, H., Tischkowitz, M., Turnbull, C., Side, L. (2018). Consensus for genes to be included on cancer panel tests offered by UK genetics services: Guidelines of the UK Cancer Genetics Group. *J. Med. Genet.*, 55(6), 1–6.

Yamauchi, H. and Takei, J. (2017). Management of hereditary breast and ovarian cancer. *Int. J. Clin. Oncol.*, 23(1), 45–51.

Endocrine neoplasia

Carling, T. (2005). Multiple endocrine neoplasia syndrome: Genetic basis for clinical management. *Curr. Opin. Oncol.*, 17, 7–12.

Christakis, I., Qiu, W., Hyde, S.M., Cote, G.J., Grubbs, E.G., Perrier, N.D., Lee, J.E. (2018). Genotype-phenotype pancreatic neuroendocrine tumor relationship in multiple endocrine neoplasia type 1 patients: A 23-year experience at a single institution. *Surgery*, 163(1), 212–217.

De Oliveira, F.M., Maeda, S.S., Marone, M.M.S., Hilário, L.N., Pagan, M.R., Colaiacovo, R., Kavabata, N.K., de Moricz, A., Medeiros Fracassi, M.T., Oliveira Hoff, A., Lourenço Júnior, D.M., Scalissi, N.M., Lima Júnior, J.V. (2017). Metastatic pancreatic gastrinoma, severe primary hyperparathyroidism, and adrenal cushing syndrome in a patient with multiple endocrine neoplasia type 1: An unusual presentation and review of the literature. *AACE Clin. Case Reports*, 3, 59–65.

Else, T. and Fishbein, L. (2018). Discovery of new susceptibility genes: Proceed cautiously. *Genet. Med.*, 20(12), 1512–1514.

Eng, C., Clayton, D., Schuffenecker, I., Lenoir, G., Cote, G., Gagel, R.F., van Amstel, H.K., Lips, C.J., Nishisho, I., Takai, S.I., March, D.J., Robinson, B.G., Frank-Raue, K., Raue, F., Xue, F., Noll, W.W., Romei, C., Pacini, F., Fink, M., Niederle, B., Zedenius, J., Nordenskjöld, M., Komminoth, P., Hendy, G.N., Mulligan, L.M. (1996). The relationship between specific RET proto-oncogene mutations and disease phenotype in multiple endocrine neoplasia type 2. *JAMA*, 276(19), 1575–1579.

Falchetti, A. (2017). Genetics of multiple endocrine neoplasia type 1 syndrome: What's new and what's old. F1000Research [Online]. Available at: https://doi.org/10.12688/f1000research.7230.1.

Foulkes, W.D., Foulkes, W.D., Bertherat, J., Eng, C., Hawking, S. (2018). 65 years of the double helix. It's all in the DNA: Understanding and managing endocrine neoplasms. *Endocrine-related Cancer*, 25(8), 8–10.

Giusti, F., Cianferotti, L., Boaretto, F., Cetani, F., Cioppi, F., Colao, A., Davì, M.V., Faggiano, A., Fanciulli, G., Ferolla, P. (2017). Multiple endocrine neoplasia syndrome type 1: Institution, management, and data analysis of a nationwide multicenter patient database. *Endocrine*, 58(2), 349–59.

Kao, S.T., Capua, C.J., Abdelsayed, R.A. (2018). Multiple endocrine neoplasia type 2b (MEN2B) in a 9-year-old female. *J. Oral Maxillofac. Surg.*, 76, 1925–1928.

Moodley, S., Weber, F., Mulligan, L.M. (2018). The evolving clinical, genetic and therapeutic landscape of multiple endocrine neoplasia type 2. *Endocrine-related Cancer*, 25(2), E1–E4.

Mucha, L., Leidig-Bruckner, G., Frank-Raue, K., Bruckner, T., Kroiss, M., Raue, F. (2017). Phaeochromocytoma in multiple endocrine neoplasia type 2: RET codon-specific pene-trance and changes in management during the last four decades. *Clin. Endocrinol.*, 87(4), 320–326.

Newey, P.J. (2017). Multiple endocrine neoplasia. *Endocrine Cancer*, 45(9), 538–542.

Plaza-menacho, I. (2017). Structure and function of RET in multiple endocrine neoplasia type 2. *Endocrine-related Cancer*, 25(2), 1–31.

Raue, F. and Frank-Raue, K. (2009). Genotype-phenotype relationship in multiple endocrine neoplasia type 2: Implications for clinical management. *Hormones*, 8(1), 23–28.

Wasserman, J.D., Tomlinson, G.E., Druker, H., Kamihara, J., Kohlmann, W.K., Kratz, C.P., Nathanson, K.L., Pajtler, K.W., Parareda, A., Rednam, S.P., States, L.J., Villani, A., Walsh, M.F., Zelley, K., Schiffman, J.D. (2017). Multiple endocrine neoplasia and hyperparathyroid-jaw tumor syndromes: Clinical features, genetics, and surveillance recommendations in childhood. *Clin. Cancer Res.*, 23(13), e123–e132.

Familial adenomatous polyposis

Aretz, S. and Nielsen, M. (2018). Adenomatous polyposis syndromes: Unexplained colorectal adenomatous polyposis. In *Hereditary Colorectal Cancer*, Valle, L., Gruber, S., Capella, G. (eds). Springer, Berlin, 161–164.

Das, V., Kalita, J., Pal, M. (2017). Predictive and prognostic biomarkers in colorectal cancer: A systematic review of recent advances and challenges. *Biomed. Pharmacother.*, 87, 8–19.

Kanth, P., Grimmett, J., Champine, M., Burt, R., Samadder, N.J. (2017). Hereditary colorectal polyposis and cancer syndromes: A primer on diagnosis and management. *Am. J. Gastroenterol.*, 112(10), 1509–1525.

Kantor, M., Sobrado, J., Patel, S., Eiseler, S., Ochner, C. (2017). Hereditary colorectal tumors: A literature review on MUTYH-associated polyposis. *Gastroenterol. Res. Pract.* 2017, 2–6.

Lorans, M., Dow, E., Macrae, F.A., Winship, I.M., Buchanan, D.D. (2018). Update on hereditary colorectal cancer: Improving the clinical utility of multigene panel testing. *Clin. Colorectal Cancer*, 17, 293–305.

Neffa, F., Garcia, L., Della Valle, A., Carusso, F., Vergara, C., Sanchez, D., Sapone, M., Silveyra, N., Revello, A.L., Esperon, P. (2018). Aggressive mutation in a familial adenomatous polyposis syndrome family: When phenotype guides clinical surveillance. *Journal of Gastrointestinal Oncology*, 9(3), 553–559.

Nielsen, M. and Aretz, S. (2018). Familial adenomatous polyposis or APC-associated polyposis. In *Hereditary Colorectal Cancer*, Valle, L., Gruber, S.B., Capellá, G. (eds). Springer, Berlin, 99–111.

Rex, D.K., Boland, C.R., Dominitz, J.A., Giardiello, F.M., Johnson, D.A., Kaltenbach, T., Levin, T.R., Lieberman, D., Robertson, D.J. (2017). Colorectal cancer screening: Recommendations for physicians and patients from the U.S. Multi-Society Task Force on colorectal cancer. *GIE*, 112, 1016–1030.

Roncucci, L., Pedroni, M., Mariani, F. (2017). Attenuated adenomatous polyposis of the large bowel: Present and future. *World. J. Gastroenterol.*, 23(23), 4135–4139.

Sample, D.C., Jewel Samadder, N., Pappas, L.M., Boucher, K.M., Samowitz, W.S., Berry, T., Westover, M., Nathan, D., Kanth, P., Byrne, K.R., Burt, R.W., Neklason, D.W. (2018). Variables affecting penetrance of gastric and duodenal phenotype in familial adenomatous polyposis patients. *BMC Gastroenterology*, 18(1), 1–8.

Talseth-Palmer, B.A. (2017). The genetic basis of colonic adenomatous polyposis syndromes. *Hereditary Cancer in Clinical Practice*, 15, 1–7.

Thomas, H. and Tomlinson, I. (2018). Hereditary mixed polyposis syndrome. In *Hereditary Colorectal Cancer*, Valle, L., Gruber, S.B., Capellá, G. (eds). Springer, Berlin, 185–192.

Valle, L. (2017). Perspectives in clinical gastroenterology and hepatology. Recent discoveries in the genetics of familial colorectal cancer and polyposis. *Clin. Gastroenterol. Hepatol.*, 15, 809–819.

Weren, R.D., Ligtenberg, M.J.L., Kets, C.M., de Voer, E.T.P., Spruijt, L., van Zelst-Stams, W.A.G., Jongmans, M.C., Glissen, C., Hehir-Kwa, J.Y., Hoischen, A., Shendure, J., Boyle, E.A., Kamping, E.J., Nagtegaal, I.D., Tops, B.B.J., Nagengast, F.M., Geurts van Kessel, A. (2015). A germline homozygous mutation in the base-excision repair gene NTHL1 causes adenomatous polyposis and colorectal cancer. *Nat. Genet.*, 47, 668–671.

Weren, R.D., Ligtenberg, M.J., Geurts van Kessel, A., de Voer, R.M., Hoogerbrugge, N., Kuiper, R.P. (2018). NTHL1 and MUTYH polyposis syndromes: Two sides of the same coin? *J. Pathol.*, 244(2), 135–142.

Familial malignant melanoma

Bassolia, S., Pellegrinid, C., Longoa, C., Di Nardod, L., Farnetania, F., Cesinarob, A.M., Pellacania, G., Concetta Fargnolid, M. (2018). Clinical, dermoscopic, and confocal features of nevi and melanomas in a multiple primary melanoma patient with the MITF p.E318Khomozygous mutation. *Melanoma Research*, 28(2), 166–169.

Bosserhoff, A. and Strizzi, L. (2017). Clinicopathologic overview of melanoma. In *Melanoma Development*, Bosserhoff, A. (ed.). Springer, Berlin.

Brown, K.M., MacGregor, S., Law, M.H. (2018). Inherited contributions to melanoma risk. In *Melanoma*, Fisher, D., Bastian, B. (eds). Springer, New York.

Chan, A.K., Han, S.J., Choy, W., Beleford, D., Aghi, M.K., Berger, M.S., Shieh, J.T., Bollen, A.W., Perry, A., Phillips, J.J., Butowski, N., Solomon, D.A. (2017). Familial melanoma-astrocytoma syndrome: Synchronous diffuse astrocytoma and pleomorphic xanthoastrocytoma in a patient with germline CDKN2A/B deletion and a significant family history. *Clin. Neuropathol.*, 36, 213–221.

Cossu, A., Casula, M., Cesaraccio, R., Lissia, A., Colombino, M., Sini, M.C., Budroni, M., Tanda, F., Paliogiannis, P., Palmieri, G. (2016). Epidemiology and genetic susceptibility of malignant melanoma in North Sardinia, Italy. *European Journal of Cancer Prevention*, 26(3), 263–267.

Cust, A.E., Mishra, K., Berwick, M. (2018). Melanoma–Role of the environment and genetics. *Photochem. Photobiol. Sci.*, 17(12), 1853–1860.

Gironi, L.C., Colombo, E., Pasini, B., Giorgione, R., Farinelli, P., Zottarelli, F., Esposto, E., Zavattaro, E., Allara, E., Ogliara, P., Betti, M., Dianzani, I., Savoia, P. (2018). Melanoma-prone families: New evidence of distinctive clinical and histological features of melanomas in CDKN2A mutation carriers. *Arch. Dermatol. Res.*, 310(10), 769–784.

Goldstein, A.M., Xiao, Y., Sampson, J., Zhu, B., Rotunno, M., Bennett, H, Wen, Y., Jones, K., Vogt, A., Burdette, L., Luo, W., Yaeger, M., Hicks, B., Han, J., De Vivo, I., Koutros, S., Andreotti, G., Beane-Freeman, L., Purdue, M., Freedman, N.D., Chanock, S.J., Tucker, M.A., Yang, X.R. (2017). Rare germline variants in known melanoma susceptibility genes in familial melanoma. *Human Molecular Genetics*, 26(24), 4886–4895.

Haugh, A.M., Njauw, C.-N., Bubley, J.A., Verzì, A.E., Zhang, B., Kudalkar, E., Van den Boom, T., Walton, K., Swick, B.L., Kumar, R., Rana, H.Q., COchrane, S., McCormick, S.R., Shea, C.R., Tsao, H., Gerami, P. (2017). Genotypic and phenotypic features of BAP1 cancer syndrome: A report of 8 new families and review of cases in the literature. *JAMA Dermatol.*, 153(10), 999–1006.

Johnson, M.M., Leachman, S.A., Aspinwall, L.G., Cranmer, L.D., Curiel-Lewandrowski, C., Sondak, V.K., Stemwedel, C.E., Swetter, S.M., Vetto, J., Bowles, T., *et al.* (2017). Skin cancer screening: Recommendations for data-driven screening guidelines and a review of the US Preventive Services Task Force controversy. *Melanoma Manag.*, 4, 13–37.

Kosmidis, C., Baka, S., Sapalidis, K., Mixalopoulos, N., Atmatzidis, S., Koulouris, H., Anthimidis, G., Varsamis, N., Zarogoulidis, P., Man, Y.-G., Georgakoudi, E., Mantalovas, S., Koimtzis, G., Tsakalidis, A., Kesisoglou, I. (2017). Melanoma from molecular pathways to clinical treatment: An up to date review. *J. Biomed.*, 2, 94–100.

Lai, V., Cranwell, W., Rodney, S. (2017). Epidemiology of skin cancer in the mature patient. *Clin. Dermatol.*, 36(2), 167–176.

Le-Shan Wilson, T., Hattangady, N., Marcondes Lerario, A., Williams, C., Koeppe, E, Quinonez, S., Osborne, J., Cha, K.B., Else, T. (2017). A new POT1 germline mutation–Expanding the spectrum of POT1-associated cancers. *Familial Cancer*, 16(4), 561–566.

Leachman, S.A., Lucero, O.M., Sampson, J.E., Cassidy, P., Bruno, W., Queirolo, P., Ghiorzo, P. (2017). Identification, genetic testing, and management of hereditary melanoma. *Cancer and Metastasis Reviews*, 36, 77–90.

Leclerc, J., Ballotti, R., Bertolotto, C. (2017). Pathways from senescence to melanoma: Focus on MITF sumoylation. *Nature Publishing Group*, 4, 1–9.

Leonardi, G.C., Falzone, L., Salemi, R., Zanghì, A., Spandidos, D.A., Mccubrey, J.A., Candido, S., Libra, M. (2018). Cutaneous melanoma: From pathogenesis to therapy (review). *Int. J. Oncol.*, 52(4), 1071–1080.

Merkel, E.A. and Gerami, P. (2017). Pathobiology in focus. Malignant melanoma of sun-protected sites: A review of clinical, histological, and molecular features. *Lab. Invest.*, 7, 1–6.

Moran, B., Silva, R., Perry, A.S., Gallagher, W.M. (2018). Epigenetics of malignant melanoma. *Seminars in Cancer Biology*, 51, 80–88.

Prasad, M.D., Rao, B.A.R., Saikumar, P. (2017). A study on malignant melanoma. *Int. J. Curr. Microbiol. App. Sci.*, 6(2), 1069–1079.

Pritchard, A.L., Johansson, P.A., Nathan, V., Howlie, M., Symmons, J., Palmer, J.M, Hayward, N.K. (2018). Germline mutations in candidate predisposition genes in individuals with cutaneous melanoma and at least two independent additional primary cancers. *PLoS One*, 13(4), 1–19.

Rai, K., Pilarski, R., Boru, G., Rehman, M., Saqr, A.H., Massengill, J.B., Singh, A., Marino, M.J., Davidorf, F.H., Cebulla, C.M., Abdel-Rahman, M.H. (2016). Germline BAP1 alterations in familial uveal melanoma. *Genes Chromosomes Cancer*, 56(2), 168–174.

Watts, C.G., Madronio, C., Morton, R.L., Goumas, C., Armstrong, B.K., Curtin, A., Menzies, S.W., Mann, G.J., Thompson, J.F., Cust, A.E. (2017). Clinical features associated with individuals at higher risk of melanoma: A population-based study. *JAMA Dermatol.*, 153(1), 23–29.

Gorlin syndrome

Akbari, M., Chen, H., Guo, G., Legan, Z., Ghali, G. (2018). Pathophysiology basal cell nevus syndrome (Gorlin syndrome): Genetic insights, diagnostic challenges, and unmet milestones. *Pathophysiology*, 25, 77–82.

Evans, D.G., Oudit, D., Smith, M.J., Rutkowski, D., Allan, E., Newman, W.G., Lear, J.T. (2017). First evidence of genotype-phenotype correlations in Gorlin syndrome. *J. Med. Genet.*, 54(8), 1–6.

Foulkes, W.D., Kamihara, J., Evans, D.G.R., Brugières, L., Bourdeaut, F., Molenaar, J.J., Walsh, M.F., Brodeur, G.M., Diller, L. (2017). Cancer surveillance in Gorlin syndrome and rhabdoid tumor predisposition syndrome. *Clinical Cancer Research*, 23, 62–68.

Ogden, T., Higgins, S., Elbaum, D., Wysong, A. (2018). The relevance of a suppressor of fused (SUFU) mutation in the diagnosis and treatment of Gorlin syndrome. *JAAD Case Reports*, 4, 196–199.

Onodera, S., Saito, A., Hasegawa, D., Morita, N., Watanabe, K., Nomura, T., Shibahara, T., Ohba, S., Yamaguchi, A., Azuma, T. (2017). Multi-layered mutation in hedgehog-related genes in Gorlin syndrome may affect the phenotype. *PLoS One*, 12(9), 1–14.

Scollon, S., Anglin, A.K., Thomas, M., Turner, J.T. (2017). A comprehensive review of pediatric tumors and associated cancer predisposition syndromes. *Journal of Genetic Counseling*, 26(3), 387–434.

Shih, S., Dai, C., Ansari, A., Urso, B.A., Laughlin, A.I., Solomon, J.A. (2018). Advances in genetic understanding of Gorlin syndrome and emerging treatment options. *Expert Opin. Orphan Drugs*, 6, 413–423.

Sosuan, G.M.N. and Chacon, A.C. (2018). Gorlin-Goltz syndrome: A rare potentially malignant disease. *International Journal of Case Reports and Images*, 1, 1–5.

Utine, G.E., Alanay, Y., Aktaş, D., Boduroğlu, K., Alikaşifoğlu, M., Tunçbilek, E. (2017). Gorlin syndrome in eleven patients/on Bir Hastada Gorlin Sendromu. *The Journal of Pediatric Research*, 4(24), 63–67.

Witmanowski, H., Szychta, P., Błochowiak, K., Jundziłł, A., Czajkowski, R. (2017). Basal cell nevus syndrome (Gorlin-Goltz syndrome): Genetic predisposition, clinical picture and treatment. *Postepy Dermatol. Alergol.*, 34(4), 9–11.

Wolkow, N., Jakobiec, F.A., Yoon, M.K., Seregard, S. (2017). Intratarsal keratinous eyelid cysts in Gorlin syndrome: A review and reappraisal. *Surv. Ophthalmol.*, 63, 711–718.

Hereditary pheochromocytoma and paraganglioma

Alfara, J.J.F., López-Rodó, L.M., Ferrández, H., Guirao, A. (2017). Recurrent spontaneous pneumothorax as a manifestation of Birt-Hogg-Dubé syndrome. *Arch. Bronconeumol.*, 54(7), 8–9.

Amorim-Pires, D., Peixoto, J., Lima, J. (2017). Hypoxia pathway mutations in pheochromocytomas and paragangliomas. *Cytogenet. Genome Res.*, 150(3–4), 227–241.

Babic, B. and Nilubol, N. (2017). Genetics of pheochromocytoma. In *Management of Adrenal Masses in Children and Adults*, Kebebew, E. (ed.). Springer, Berlin, 85–103.

Bholah, R. and Bunchman, T.E. (2017). Review of pediatric pheochromocytoma and paragan-glioma. *Front. Pediatr.*, 5, 1–14.

Crona, J., Ta, D., Pacak, K. (2017). New perspectives on pheochromocytoma and paraganglioma: Toward a molecular classification. *Endocr. Rev.*, 38(6), 489–515.

Ganeshan, D. and Kundra, V. (2017). The ABCs of BHD: An in-depth review of Birt-Hogg-Dubé syndrome. *AJR Am. J. Roentgenol.*, 209(6), 1291–1296.

Geilswijk, M., Bendstrup, E., Gebauer, M. (2018). Skytte MSA. Childhood pneumothorax in Birt-Hogg-Dubé syndrome: A cohort study and review of the literature. *Mol. Genet. Genomic Med.*, 6(3), 332–338.

Hamidi, O., Young Jr., W.F., Iñiguez-Ariza, N.M., Kittah, N.E., Gruber, L., Bancos, C., Tamhane, S., Bancos, I. (2017). Malignant pheochromocytoma and paraganglioma: 272 patients over 55 years. *J. Clin. Endocrinol. Metab.*, 102(9), 3296–3305.

Jochmanova, I., Wolf, K.I., King, K.S., Nambuba, J., Wesley, R., Martucci, V., Raygada, M., Adams, K.T., Prodanov, T., Tito Fojo, A., Luzurova, I., Pacak, K. (2017). Genomic landscape of pheochromocytoma and paraganglioma. *Trends Cancer*, 4(1), 6–9.

Khatami, F. and Tavangar, S.M. (2017). Current diagnostic status of pheochromocytomaand future perspective: A mini review. *J. Pathol.*, 12(3), 313–322.

Lenders, J.W.M. and Eisenhofer, G. (2017). Update on modern management of pheochromo-cytoma and paraganglioma. *Endocrinol. Metab.*, 32(2), 152–161.

Pereira, B.D., da Silva, T.N., Bernardo, A.T., César, R., Luiz, H.V., Pacak, K., Mota-Vieira, L. (2018). A clinical roadmap to investigate the genetic basis of pediatric pheochromocytoma: Which genes should physicians think about? *International Journal of Endocrinology*, 2018.

Rednam, S.P., Erez, A., Druker, H., Janeway, K.A., Kamihara, J., Kohlmann, W.K., Nathanson, K.L., States, L.J., Tomlinson, G.E., Villani, A., Voss, S.D., Schiffman, J.D., Wasserman, J.D. (2017). von Hippel–Lindau and hereditary pheochromocytoma/paraganglioma syndromes: Clinical features, genetics, and surveillance recommendations in childhood. *Clin. Cancer Res.*, (12)23, 68–76.

Rijken, J.A., Niemeijer, N.D., Jonker, M.A., Eijkelenkamp, K., Jansen, J.C., van Berkel, A., Timmers, H.J.L.M., Kunst, H.P.M., Bisschop, P.H.L.T., Kerstens, M.N., Dreijerink, K.M.A., van Dooren, M.F., van ders Horst-Schrivers, A.N.A., Hes, F.J., Leemans, C.R., Corssmit, E.P.M., Hensen, E.F. (2017). The penetrance of paraganglioma and pheochromocytoma in SDHB germline mutation carriers. *Clin. Genet.*, 91(1), 60–66.

Ripperger, T., Bielack, S.S., Borkhardt, A., Brecht, I.B., Burkhardt, B., Calaminus, G., Debatin, K.-M., Deubzer, H., Dirksen, U., Eckert, C. *et al.* (2017). Childhood cancer predisposition syndromes – A concise review and recommendations by the Cancer Predisposition Working Group of the Society for Pediatric Oncology and Hematology. *Am. J. Med. Genet. A.*, 173(4), 1–21.

Schmidt, L.S. and Linehan, W.M. (2017). PT US CR. FLCN: The causative gene for Birt-Hogg-Dubé syndrome. *Gene*, 640, 28–42.

Scollon, S., Anglin, A.K., Thomas, M., Turner, J.T. (2017). A comprehensive review of pediatric tumors and associated cancer predisposition syndromes. *Journal of Genetic Counseling*, 26(3), 387–434.

Toledo, R. and Jimenez, C. (2018). Recent advances in the management of malignant pheochromocytoma and paraganglioma: Focus on tyrosine kinase and hypoxia-inducible factor inhibitors [Online]. Available at: https://f1000research.com/articles/7-1148/v1.

Tong, Y., Schneider, J.A., Coda, A.B., Hata, T.R. (2018). Syndrome: A review of dermatological Birt-Hogg-Dubé manifestations and other symptoms. *Am. J. Clin. Dermatol.*, 19, 87–101.

Turchini, J., Gill, A.J., Tischler, A.S. (2018). Pathology of pheochromocytoma and paraganglioma. *Histopathology*, 72(1), 97–105.

Infracentesimal syndromes

Alter, B.P., Giri, N., Savage, S.A., Rosenberg, P.S. (2018). Cancer in the National Cancer Institute inherited bone marrow failure syndrome cohort after fifteen years of follow-up. *Correspondence*, 103, 30–39.

Beckers, A., Petrossians, P., Hanson, J., Daly, A.F. (2018). The causes and consequences of pituitary gigantism. *Nat. Rev. Endocrinol.*, 14, 705–720.

Belén, M., Schamun, B., Correa, R., Graffigna, P., de Miguel, V., Fainstein, P. (2018). Endocrinología, Diabetes y Nutrición Carney complex review: Genetic features. *Endocrinol. Diabetes y Nutr.*, 65, 52–59.

Bouman, A., Van Koningsbruggen, S., Karakullukcu, M.B., Schreuder, W.H., Lakeman, P. (2018). Bloom syndrome does not always present with sun-sensitive facial erythema. *Eur. J. Med. Genet.*, 61(2), 94–97.

Brosh Jr., R.M., Bellani, M., Liu, Y., Seidman, M.M. (2017). Fanconi anemia: A DNA repair disorder characterized by accelerated decline of the hematopoietic stem cell compartment and other features of aging. *Ageing Res. Rev.*, 33, 67–75.

Campbell, M.B., Campbell, W.C., Rogers, J., Rogers, N., Rogers, Z., van den Hurk, A.M., Webb, A., Webb, T., Zaslaw, P. (2018). Bloom syndrome: Research and data priorities for the development of precision medicine as identified by some affected families. *Cold Spring Harb. Mol. Case Stud.*, 4(2), 1–12.

Chintalacheruvu, L.M., Shaw, T., Buddam, A., Diab, O., Kassim, T., Mukherjee, S. (2017). Major hereditary gastrointestinal cancer syndromes: A narrative review. *J. Gastrointestin. Liver Dis.*, 26, 157–163.

Cunniff, C., Bassetti, A., Ellis, N.A. (2017). Bloom's syndrome: Clinical spectrum, molecular pathogenesis, and cancer predisposition. *Molecular Syndromology*, 8(1), 4–23.

Daly, A.F. and Beckers, A. (2017). Genetics of pituitary tumor syndromes. In *The Pituitary, 4th edition*, Shlomo, M. (ed.). Academic Press, 619–630.

De Silva, G.S., Lairmore, T.C., Moley, J.F. (2017). Familial Hyperparathyroidism: Multiple Endocrine Neoplasia Types II and I; Familial Hypocalciuric Hypercalcemia; Hyperparathyroidism-Jaw Tumor Syndrome. In *Medical and Surgical Treatment of Parathyroid Diseases*. Springer, Cham, 57–68.

Dimaras, H. and Corson, T.W. (2018). Retinoblastoma, the visible CNS tumor: A review. *J. Neurosci. Res.*, 97(1), 29–44.

Fabian, I.D., Onadim, Z., Karaa, E., Duncan, C., Chowdhury, T., Scheimberg, I. (2018). The management of retinoblastoma. *Oncogene*, 37(12), 1551–1560.

Feurstein, S. and Godley, L.A. (2017). Germline ETV6 mutations and predisposition to hematological malignancies. *Int. J. Hematol.*, 106(2), 189–195.

Furutani, E. and Shimamura, A. (2017). Germline genetic predisposition to hematologic malignancy. *J. Clin. Oncol.*, 35(9), 1018–1028.

Ganeshan, D., Menias, C.O., Pickhardt, P.J., Sandrasegaran, K., Lubner, M.G., Ramalingam, P., Bhalla, S. (2018). Tumors in von Hippel–Lindau syndrome: From head to toe – Comprehensive state-of-the-art review. *RadioGraphics*, 38(3), 849–866.

Gaur, S., Turkbey, B., Choyke, P. (2017). Hereditary renal tumor syndromes: Update on diagnosis and management. *Semin. Ultrasound CT*, 38(1), 59–71.

Godley, L.A. and Shimamura, A. (2018). Genetic predisposition to hematologic malignancies: Management and surveillance. *Blood, The Journal of the American Society of Hematology*, 130, 424–433.

Guidugli, L., Johnson, A.K., Alkorta-Aranburu, G., Nelakuditi, V., Arndt, K., Churpek, J.E., Godley, L.A., Townsley, D., Young, N.S., Fitzpatrick, C., del Gaudio, D., Das, S., Li, Z. (2017). Clinical utility of gene panel-based testing for hereditary myelodysplastic syndrome/acute leukemia predisposition syndromes. *Leukemia*, 31(5), 1226–1229.

Hansen-Kiss, E., Beinkampen, S., Adler, B., Frazier, T., Prior, T., Erdman, S., Eng, C. and Herman, G. (2017). A retrospective chart review of the features of PTEN hamartoma tumour syndrome in children. *J. Med. Genet.*, 54(7), 1–8.

Jerzak, K.J., Mancuso, T., Eisen, A. (2018). Ataxia–telangiectasia gene (ATM) mutation heterozygosity in breast cancer: A narrative review. *Curr. Oncol.*, 25, 176–180.

Kamihara, J., Bourdeaut, F., Foulkes, W.D., Molenaar, J.J., Mossé, Y.P., Nakagawara, A., Parareda, A., Scollon, S.R., Schneider, K.W., Skalet, A.H., States, L.J., Walsh, M.F., Diller, L.R., Brodeur, G.M. (2017). Retinoblastoma and neuroblastoma predisposition and surveillance. *Clin. Cancer Res.*, 23, 98–107.

Lehmann, A.R., Mcgibbon, D., Stefanini, M. (2011). Xeroderma pigmentosum. *Orphanet J. Rare Dis.*, 6, 70.

Liu, Q., Tong, D., Liu, G., Yi, Y., Zhang, D., Zhang, J., Zhang, Y., Huang, Z., Li, Y., Chen, R., Guan, Y., Yi, X., Jiang, J. (2017). Carney complex with PRKAR1A gene mutation: A case report and literature review. *Medicine*, 96, 1–4.

Maher, E.R. (2018). Hereditary renal cell carcinoma syndromes: Diagnosis, surveillance and management. *World J. Urol.*, 36, 1891–1898.

Mamrak, N.E., Shimamura, A., Howlett, N.G. (2017). Recent discoveries in the molecular pathogenesis of the inherited bone marrow failure syndrome Fanconi anemia. *Blood Reviews*, 31(3), 93–99.

Mangray, S. (2018). Heritable forms of primary hyperparathyroidism: A current perspective. *Histopathology*, 72(1), 117–132.

Moriwaki, S., Kanda, F., Hayashi, M., Yamashita, D. (2017). Xeroderma pigmentosum clinical practice guidelines. *The Journal of Dermatology*, 125, 2013–2022.

Ngeow, J., Courtney, E., Lim, K.H., Eng, C. (2018). Hamartomatous polyposis syndromes. In *Hereditary Colorectal Cancer*, Valle, L., Gruber, S.B., Capellá, G. (eds). Springer, Berlin.

Oshima, J., Sidorova, J.M., Monnat, R.J. (2017). Werner syndrome: Clinical features, pathogenesis and potential therapeutic interventions. *Ageing Res. Rev.*, 33, 105–114.

Pinkson, S. (2017). General pituitary disorders. *Physician Assistant Clinics*, 2(1), 107-122.

Rostomyan, L., Potorac, I., Beckers, P., Daly, A.F., Beckers, A. (2017). AIP mutations and gigantism. *Ann. Endocrinol.*, 78, 123–130.

Saida, S. (2017). Predispositions to leukemia in Down syndrome and other hereditary disorders. *Curr. Treat. Options in Oncol.* 18, 41.

Savage, S.A. and Walsh, M.F. (2018). Myelodysplastic syndrome, acute myeloid leukemia, and cancer surveillance in Fanconi anemia. *Hematol. Clin.*, 32, 657–668.

Shamanna, R.A., Croteau, D.L., Lee, J., Bohr, V.A. (2017). Recent advances in understanding Werner syndrome, *F1000Research*, 6, 1–12.

Shiloh, Y. and Lederman, H.M. (2017). Ataxia-telangiectasia (A-T): An emerging dimension of premature ageing. *Ageing Res. Rev.*, 33, 76–88.

Strand, M.S., Lockhart, A.C., Fields, R.C. (2017). Genetics of gastric cancer. *Surg. Clin.*, 97, 345–370.

Stratakis, C.A. and Carney, J.A. (2017). Cushing syndrome in Carney complex: Clinical, pathological, and molecular genetic findings in the 17 affected Mayo clinic patients. *The American Journal of Surgical Pathology*, 41(2), 171–181.

Valdez, J.M., Nichols, K.E., Kesserwan, C. (2017). Li-Fraumeni syndrome: A paradigm for the understanding of hereditary cancer predisposition. *Br. J. Haematol.*, 176(4), 539–552.

Varshney, N., Kebede, A.A., Owusu-Dapaah, H., Lather, J., Kaushik, M., Bhullar, J.S. (2017). A review of von Hippel-Lindau syndrome. *J. Kidney Cancer VHL*, 4(3), 20–29.

Villani, A., Shore, A., Wasserman, J.D., Stephens, D., Kim, R.H., Druker, H., Gallinger, B., Naumer, A., Kohlmann, W., Novokmet, A., Tabori, U., Tijerin, M., Greer, M.-L.C., Finlay, J.L., Schiffman, J.D., Malkin, D. (2016). Biochemical and imaging surveillance in germline TP53 mutation carriers with Li-Fraumeni syndrome: 11 year follow-up of a prospective observational study. *Lancet. Oncol.*, 17, 1295–1305.

Walsh, M.F., Chang, V.Y., Kohlmann, W.K., Scott, H.S., Cunniff, C., Bourdeaut, F., Molenaar, J.J., Porter, C.C., Sandlund, J.T., Plon, S.E., Wang, L.L., Savage, S.A. (2017). Recommendations for childhood cancer screening and surveillance in DNA repair disorders. *Clin. Cancer Res.*, 23(11), 23–32.

Zaanan, A., Bouché, O., Benhaim, L., Buecher, B., Chapelle, N., Dubreuil, O., Fares, N., Granger, V., Lefort, C., Gagniere, J., Meilleroux, J., Baumann, A.-S., Vendrely, V., Ducreux, M., Michel, P. (2018). Gastric cancer: French intergroup clinical practice guidelines for diagnosis, treatments and follow-up. *Dig. Liver Dis.*, 50, 768–779.

Zhang, H., Feng, M., Feng, Y., Bu, Z., Li, Z., Jia, S., Ji, J. (2018). Germline mutations in hereditary diffuse gastric cancer. *Chin. J. Cancer Res.*, 30, 122–130.

Lynch syndrome

Aissaoui, S., Cartellier, C., Seytier, T., Giraud, S., Calender, A. (2017). Calcul du risque de mutation génétique dans le cadre du syndrome de Lynch : évaluation de l'utilité du logiciel PREMM1.2.6 à Lyon : 1re étude française. *Bull. Cancer. Société française du cancer*, 104, 288–294.

Blount, J. and Prakash, A. (2018). The changing landscape of Lynch syndrome due to PMS2 mutations. *Clin. Genet.*, 94, 61–69.

Bujanda, L. and Herreros-Villanueva, M. (2017). Pancreatic cancer in lynch syndrome patients. *J. Cancer*, 8, 3667–3674.

Burke, W.M., Orr, J., Leitao, M., Salom, E., Gehrig, P., Olawaiye, A.B., Brewer, M., Boruta, D., Villella, J., Herzog, T., Abu Shahin, F. (2014a). Endometrial cancer: A review and current management strategies: Part I. *Gynecol. Oncol.*, 134, 385–392.

Burke, W.M., Orr, J., Leitao, M., Salom, E., Gehrig, P., Olawaiye, A.B., Brewer, M., Boruta, D., Villella, J., Herzog, T., Abu Shahin, F. (2014b). Endometrial cancer: A review and current management strategies: Part II. *Gynecol. Oncol.*, 134, 393–402.

Cox, V.L., Bamashmos, A.A.S., Yedururi, S. (2018). Lynch syndrome: Genomics update and imaging review 1. *Radiographics*, 38(2), 483–499.

Davies, H., Morganella, S., Purdie, C.A., Jang, S.J., Borgen, E., Russnes, H., Glodzik, D., Zou, X., Viari, A., Richardson, A.L., Børresen-Dale, A.-L., Thompson, A., Eyfjord, J.E., Kong, G., Stratton, M.R., Nik-Zainal, S. (2017). Whole-genome sequencing reveals breast cancers with mismatch repair deficiency. *Cancer Res.*, 77, 4755–4762.

Galiatsatos, P., Labos, C., Jeanjean, M., Miller, K., Foulkes, W.D. (2017). Low yield of gastroscopy in patients with Lynch syndrome. *Turkish J. Gastroenterol.*, 28(6), 434–438.

Hansen, M.F., Johansen, J., Sylvander, A.E., Bjørnevoll, I., Talseth-Palmer, B.A., Lavik, L.A.S., Xavier, A., Engebretsen, L.F., Scott, R.J., Drabløs, F., Sjursen, W. (2017). Use of multigene-panel identifies pathogenic variants in several CRC-predisposing genes in patients previously tested for Lynch syndrome. *Clin. Genet.*, 92, 405–414.

Herzig, D.O., Buie, W.D., Weiser, M.R., You, Y.N., Rafferty, J.F., Feingold, D., Steele, S.R. (2017). Clinical practice guidelines for the surgical treatment of patients with Lynch syndrome. *Dis. Colon Rectum*, 60, 137–143.

Köbel, M., Tessier-Cloutier, B., Leo, J., Hoang, L.N., Blake Gilks C., Soslow, R.A., Delair, D., Stewart, C.J.R., Lee, C.-H. (2017). Frequent mismatch repair protein deficiency in mixed endometrioid and clear cell carcinoma of the endometrium. *Int. J. Gynecol. Pathol.*, 36, 555–561.

Le, S., Ansari, U., Mumtaz, A., Malik, K., Patel, P., Doyle, A., Khachemoune, A. (2017). Lynch syndrome and Muir-Torre syndrome: An update and review on the genetics, epidemiology, and management of two related disorders. *Dermatol. Online J.*, 23.

Luba, D.G., DiSario, J.A., Rock, C., Saraiya, D., Moyes, K., Brown, K., Rushton, K., Ogara, M.M., Raphael, M., Zimmerman, D., Garrido, K., Silguero, E., Nelson, J., Yurgelun, M.B., Kastrinos, F., Wenstrup, R.J., Syngal, S. (2018). Community practice implementation of a self-administered version of $PREMM_{1,2,6}$ to assess risk for Lynch syndrome. *Clin. Gastroenterol. Hepatol.*, 16, 49–58.

Lynch, H.T. and de la Chapelle, A. (2003). Hereditary colorectal cancer. *N. Engl. J. Med.*, 348, 919–932.

Lynch, H.T., Lanspa, S., Shaw, T., Casey, M.J., Rendell, M., Stacey, M., Townley, T., Snyder, C., Hitchins, M., Bailey-Wilson, J. (2018). Phenotypic and genotypic heterogeneity of Lynch syndrome: A complex diagnostic challenge. *Fam. Cancer.*, 17, 403–414.

Malik, S.S., Lythgoe, M.P., McPhail, M., Monahan, K.J. (2017). Metachronous colorectal cancer following segmental or extended colectomy in Lynch syndrome: A systematic review and meta-analysis. *Fam. Cancer*, 17(4), 1–8.

McAlpine, J., Leon-Castillo, A., Bosse, T. (2018). The rise of a novel classification system for endometrial carcinoma; integration of molecular subclasses. *J. Pathol.*, 244, 538–549.

Møller, P., Seppälä, T.T., Bernstein, I., Holinski-Feder, E., Sala, P., Gareth Evans, D., Lindblom, A., Macrae, F., Blanco, I., Sijmons, R.F., *et al.* (2018). Cancer risk and survival in path_MMR carriers by gene and gender up to 75 years of age: A report from the prospective Lynch Syndrome Database. *Gut*, 67, 1306–1316.

NHS Health Education England (2020). Genomics Education Programme [Online]. Available at: https://www.genomicseducation.hee.nhs.uk/documents/lynch-syndrome/.

Niskakoski, A., Pasanen, A., Lassus, H., Renkonen-Sinisalo, L., Kaur, S., Mecklin, J.P., Bützow, R., Peltomäki, P. (2018). Molecular changes preceding endometrial and ovarian cancer: A study of consecutive endometrial specimens from Lynch syndrome surveillance. *Mod. Pathol.*, 31(8), 1–11.

Pearlman, R., Frankel W.L., Swanson, B., Zhao, W., Yilmaz, A., Miller, K., Bacher, J., Bigley, C., Nelsen, L., Goodfellow, P.J. *et al.* (2017). Prevalence and spectrum of germline cancer susceptibility gene mutations among patients with early-onset colorectal cancer. *JAMA Oncol.*, 3, 464–471.

Peltomäki, P. and Gylling, A. (2005). Brain tumors and the Lynch syndrome. *OAPEN*, 6, 45–50.

Phelan, A., Lopez-Beltran, A., Montironi, R., Zhang, S., Raspollini, M.R., Cheng, M., Kaimakliotis, H.Z., Koch, M.O., Cheng, L. (2018). Inherited forms of bladder cancer: A review of Lynch syndrome and other inherited conditions. *Futur. Oncol.*, 14, 277–290.

Pradere, B., Lotan, Y., Roupret, M. (2017). Lynch syndrome in upper tract urothelial carcinoma: Significance, screening, and surveillance. *Curr. Opin. Urol.*, 27, 48–55.

Ramchander, N.C., Ryan, N.A.J., Crosbie, E.J., Evans, D.G. (2017). Homozygous germ-line mutation of the PMS2 mismatch repair gene: A unique case report of constitutional mismatch repair deficiency (CMMRD). *BMC Medical Genetics*, 18, 1–8.

Razvi, M.A., Giardiello, F.M., Law, J.K. (2017). DNA mismatch repair and Lynch syndrome. *Current Colorectal Cancer Reports*, 13, 212–219.

Roberts, M.E., Jackson, S.A., Susswein, L.R., Zeinomar, N., Ma, X., Marshall, M.L., Stettner, A,R., Milewski, B., Xu, Z., Solomon, B.D., Terry, M.B., Hruska, K.S., Klein, R.T., Chung, W.K. (2018). MSH6 and PMS2 germ-line pathogenic variants implicated in Lynch syndrome are associated with breast cancer. *Genet. Med.*, 20(10), 1–8.

Ryan, N.A.J., Evans, D.G., Green, K., Crosbie, E.J. (2017a). Pathological features and clinical behavior of Lynch syndrome-associated ovarian cancer. *Gynecol. Oncol.*, 144, 491–495.

Ryan, N.A.J., Morris, J., Green, K., Lalloo, F., Woodward, E.R., Hill, J., Crosbie, E.J., Evans, D.G. (2017b). Association of mismatch repair mutation with age at cancer onset in Lynch syndrome: Implications for stratified surveillance strategies. *JAMA Oncol.*, 3, E1–E5.

Samadder, N.J., Smith, K.R., Wong, J., Thomas, A., Hanson, H., Boucher, K., Kopituch, C., Cannon-Albright, L.A., Burt, R.W., Curtin, K. (2017). Cancer risk in families fulfilling the Amsterdam criteria for Lynch syndrome. *JAMA Oncol.*, 3, 1697.

Shlien, A., Campbell, B.B., de Borja, R., Alexandrov, L.B., Merico, D., Wedge, D., Van Loo, P., Tarpey, P.S., Coupland, P., Behjati, S. *et al.* (2015). Combined hereditary and somatic mutations of replication error repair genes result in rapid onset of ultra-hypermutated cancers. *Nat. Genet.*, 47, 257–262.

de Silva, G.S., Lairmore, T.C., Moley, J.F. (2017). Familial hyperparathyroidism: Multiple endocrine neoplasia types II and I; familial hypocalciuric hypercalcemia; hyperparathyroidism-jaw tumor syndrome. In *Medical and Surgical Treatment of Parathyroid Diseases*. Springer, Berlin, 57–68.

Sloan, E.A., Ring, K.L., Willis, B.C., Modesitt, S.C., Mills, A.M. (2017). PD-L1 expression in mismatch repair-deficient endometrial carcinomas, including Lynch syndrome-associated and MLH1 promoter hypermethylated tumors. *Am. J. Surg. Pathol.*, 41, 326–333.

Therkildsen, C., Ladelund, S., Smith-Hansen, L., Lindberg, L.J., Nilbert, M. (2017). Towards gene-and gender based risk estimates in Lynch syndrome; age-specific incidences for 13 extra-colorectal cancer types. *Br. J. Cancer.*, 117, 1702–1710.

Tognetto, A., Michelazzo, M.B., Calabró, G.E., Unim, B., Di Marco, M., Ricciardi, W., Pastorino, R., Boccia, S. (2017). A systematic review on the existing screening pathways for Lynch syndrome identification. *Front. Public Heal.* 5, 1–7.

Vargas-Parra, G., Navarro, M., Pineda, M., Capellá, G. (2018). The molecular basis of Lynch-like syndrome. In *Hereditary Colorectal Cancer: Genetic Basis and Clinical Implications*, Valle L., Gruber S., Capellá G. (eds). Springer, Cham, 21–41.

Wang, T. and Fernando, E.H. (2017). Prediction of new cancer in patients with Lynch syndrome based on mutation patterns. *JAMA*, 296(12), 3–4.

Watkins, J.C., Yang, E.J., Muto, M.G., Feltmate, C.M., Berkowitz, R.S., Horowitz, N.S., (2017). Universal screening for mismatch-repair deficiency in endometrial cancers to identify patients with Lynch syndrome and Lynch-like syndrome. *Int. J. Gynecol. Pathol.*, 36, 115–127.

Wielders, E., Delzenne-Goette, E., Dekker, R., Van der Valk, M., te Riele, H. (2017). Truncation of the MSH2 C-terminal 60 amino acids disrupts effective DNA mismatch repair and is causative for Lynch syndrome. *Fam. Cancer*, 16, 221–229.

Wimmer, K., Brugières, L., Duval, A., Muleris, M., Kratz, C.P., Vasen, H.F.A. (2015). Communications: Constitutional or biallelic? Settling on a name for a recessively inherited cancer susceptibility syndrome. *J. Med. Genet.*, 53, 226.

Wimmer, K. and Etzler, J. (2008). Constitutional mismatch repair-deficiency syndrome: Have we so far seen only the tip of an iceberg? *Hum. Genet.*, 124, 105–122.

Win, A.K., Jenkins, M.A., Dowty, J.G., Antoniou, A.C., Lee, A., Giles, G.G., Buchanan, D.D., Clendenning, M., Rosty, C., Ahnen, D.J., Thibodeau, S.N., Casey, G., Gallinger, S., Le Marchand, L., Haile, R.W., Potter, J.D., Zheng, Y., Lindor, N.M., Newcomb, P.A., Hopper, J.L., MacInnis, R.J. (2017). Prevalence and penetrance of major genes and polygenes for colorectal cancer. *Cancer Epidemiol. Biomarkers Prev.*, 26, 404–412.

Neurofibromatosis

Allaway, R.J., Gosline, S.J.C., La Rosa, S., Knight, P., Bakker, A., Guinney, J., Le, L.Q. (2018). Cutaneous neurofibromas in the genomics era: Current understanding and open questions. *British Journal of Cancer*, 118, 1539–1548.

Batista, P., Goloni-Bertollo, E.M., Costa, D.D.S. (2014). Neurofibromatoses: Part 1 – Diagnosis and differential diagnosis. *Arq. Neuropsiquiatr.*, 72(3), 241–250.

Castellanos, E., Plana, A., Carrato, C., Carrió, M., Rosas, I., Amilibia, E., Roca-Ribas, F., Hostalot, C., Castillo, A., Ros, A., Quer, A., Becerra, J.L., Salvador, H., Lázaro, C., Blanco, I., Serra, E., Bielsa, I. (2018). Early genetic diagnosis of neurofibromatosis type 2 from skin plaque plexiform schwannomas in childhood. *JAMA Dermatol.*, 154(3), 341–346.

Jeon, Y.W., Kim, R.M., Lim, S.T., Choi, H.J., Suh, Y.J. (2015). Early-onset breast cancer in a family with neurofibromatosis type 1 associated with a germline mutation in BRCA1. *J. Breast Cancer*, 18(1), 97–100.

Kuhlen, M. (2018). Trio sequencing in pediatric cancer and clinical implications. *EMBO Mol. Med.*, 10(4), 1–7.

Leandro, M., Souza, R., Morato, E. (2015). Neurofibromatosis: Part 2 – Clinical management. *Arq. Neuropsiquiatr.*, 73(6), 531–543.

Linder, C., Smith, M.J., Bulman, A., Wallace, A., Freemont, A.J., Mangham, D.C., Evans, D.G.R. (2018). Sarcoma in neurofibromatosis 2: Case report and review of the literature. *Fam. Cancer*, 18(1), 97–100.

Lloyd, S.K.W. and Evans, D.G.R. (2013). Neurofibromatosis type 2 (NF2): Diagnosis and management. *Handb. Clin. Neurol.*, 115, 957–967.

Medical Genomics Laboratory Department of Genetics (2017). Comprehensive Testing for Neurofibromatoses, RASopathies, and Tuberous Sclerosis at UAB. Medical Genomics Laboratory, Birmingham.

Moyhuddin, A., Baser, M.E., Watson, C., Purcell, S., Ramsden, R.T., Heiberg, A., Wallace, A.J., Evans, D.G.R. (2003). Somatic mosaicism in neurofibromatosis 2: Prevalence and risk of disease transmission to offspring. *J. Med. Genet.*, 40(6), 459–463.

Plotkin, S.R. and Wick, A. (2018). Neurofibromatosis and schwannomatosis. *Semin. Neurol.*, 38(1), 73–85.

Ruggieri, M., Serra, A., Maiolino, L., Cocuzza, S., Di Mauro, P., Licciardello, L., Milone, P., Privitera, G., Belfiore, G., Di Raimondo, F., Romano, A., Charenza, A., Muglia, M., Polizzi, A., Evans, D.G. (2016). Childhood neurofibromatosis type 2 (NF2) and related disorders: From bench to bedside and biologically targeted therapies. *Acta Otorhinolaryngol. Ital.*, 36(5), 345–367.

Sato, T. and Sekido, Y. (2018). NF2/merlin inactivation and potential therapeutic targets in mesothelioma. *Int. J. Mol. Sci.*, 19(4), 988.

RASopathies

Aoki, Y., Niihori, T., Inoue, S., Matsubara, Y. (2015). Recent advances in RASopathies. *J. Hum. Genet.*, 11, 1–7.

Bessis, D. (2010). Syndromes neuro-cardio-facio-cutanés et RASopathie. *Images en dermatologie*, 3(4), 122–128.

Çelik, N., Cinaz, P., Bideci, A., Yüce, Ö., Emeksiz, H.C., Döğer, E., Çamurdan, O. (2014). Cardio-facio-cutaneous syndrome with precocious puberty, growth hormone deficiency and hyperprolactinemia. *Journal of Clinical Research in Pediatric Endocrinology*, 6(1), 55–58.

Hafner, C. and Groesser, L. (2013). Mosaic RASopathies. *Cell Cycle*, 12(1), 43–50.

Leung, G.K.C., Luk, H.M., Tang, V.H.M., Gao, W.W., Mak, C.C.Y., Yu, M.H.C., Wong, L., Chu, Y.W.Y., Yang, W.L., Wong, W.H.S., Ma, A.C.H., Leung, A.Y.H., Jin, D.Y., Chan, K.Y.K., Allanson, J., Lo, I.F.M. (2018). Integrating functional analysis in the next-generation sequencing diagnostic pipeline of RASopathies. *Sci. Rep.*, 8(1), 1–9.

Messiaen, L., Yao, S., Brems, H., Callens, T., Sathienkijkanchai, A., Denayer, E., Spencer, E., Arn, P., Babovic-Vuksanovic, D. *et al.* (2015). Clinical and mutational spectrum of neurofibromatosis type 1-like syndrome. *JAMA*, 302, 2111–2118.

Plotkin, S.R., Blakeley, J.O., Evans, D.G., Hanemann, C.O., Hulsebos, T.J.M., Hunter-Schaedle, K., Kalpana, G.V., Korf, B., Messiaen, L., Papi, L., Ratner, N., Sherman, L.S., Smith, M.J., Stemmer-Rachamimov, A.O., Vitte, J., Giovanni, M. (2014). Update from the 2011 International Schwannomatosis Workshop: From genetics to diagnostic criteria. *Am. J. Med. Genet. Part A*, 161A, 405–416.

Rauen, K.A. (2013). The RASopathies. *Annu. Rev. Genomics Hum. Genet.*, 14, 355–369.

Rauen, K.A., Huson, S.M., Burkitt-Wright, E., Evans, D.G., Farschtschi, S., Ferner, R.E., Gutmann, D.H., Hanemann, C.O., Kerr, B., Legius, E., Parada, L.F., Patton, M., Peltonen, J., Ratner, N., Riccardi, V.M., van der Vaart, T., Vikkula, M., Viskochil, D.H., Zenker, M., Upadhyaya, M. (2015). Recent developments in neurofibromatoses and RASopathies: Management, diagnosis and current and future therapeutic avenues. *American Journal of Medical Genetics Part A*, 167(1), 1–10.

Santoro, C., Pacileo, G., Limongelli, G., Scianguetta, S., Giugliano, T., Piluso, G. (2014). Leopard syndrome: Clinical dilemmas in differential diagnosis of RASopathies. *BMC Medical Genetics*, 15, 1–6.

Torrelo, A. (2011). Rasopathies: Developmental disorders that predispose to cancer and skin manifestations. *Actas Dermosifiliogr.*, 102(6), 402–416.

Villani, A., Greer, M.C., Kalish, J.M., Nakagawara, A., Nathanson, K.L., Pajtler, K.W., Walsh, M.F., Wasserman, J.D., Zelley, K., Kratz, C.P. (2017). Recommendations for cancer surveillance in individuals with RASopathies and other rare genetic conditions with increased cancer risk. *Clinic Cancer Research*, 23(12), 83–91.

Index

C

D, E

F

G, H

I, J, K

L

M

N, O

P

R

S

T

U, V

W, X